KEEPING IT UNDER WRAPS: SEX

KEEPING IT UNDER WRAPS: SEX

An Anthology

LOUISE BRYANT, TRACY HOPE, ALNAAZE NATHOO

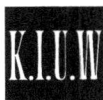

K.I.U.W

Keeping It Under Wraps

This anthology is dedicated to Clara and Liam, for tearing off the first corner.

CONTENTS

Content Warning

Some of the essays in this book include topics such as sexual violence, drug abuse, assault and other related themes.

The writers of these essays come from diverse cultural and generational backgrounds. Their voices and their views are their own.

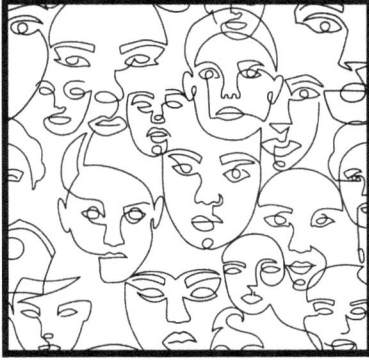

Introduction

The idea for an anthology about sex started with a group of friends talking about their sex lives over a drink one wintry evening. As we compared stories, it was clear that everyone felt different, or weird, because of their feelings about and approach to sex. Over wine and friendship, the conversation deepened. We realised that we are so brainwashed about what sex should be, what it should look like, and how it should feel, that our realities become irrelevant. Instead of living with our own reality, we have to live with what others say it should be. And when we live like that, we always come up short.

We decided to spread the word and see who felt comfortable sharing their personal experiences with us. It was a big ask, finding people willing to open up about their anxieties, their traumas, their shame, and their innermost desires. These are things we don't talk about – but shouldn't we?

This anthology brings together people from around the

world with diverse experiences and reflections on what sex and sexuality is for them. Very quickly, we saw that the stories were unique, and yet, the themes were universal.

No matter our relationships or expectations, we are all looking for joy and acceptance – a way to belong not only to our own smaller communities but also to a larger community, where who we are is normal, ok, acceptable.

We have worth and meaning. We are enough.

Sex isn't always pleasure. There is trauma, there is pain, there is inadequacy, there is shame, there is indifference. As much as we have to destigmatise pleasure, we must also not be afraid of talking about how people can inflict pain on others in the search to fulfil their own needs, fears, and expectations.

There is hope. In the saddest stories and the most traumatic experiences, sometimes the simple lesson is that right now, in this moment, it's ok to not be ok. That our experiences, our hopes, and understanding – well, it's all a bit muffled and fuzzy. Life can be shit and sex can be shit and people can be shit. That's ok.

In the end, it's about finding self-acceptance and love, especially from the most important person in your life: yourself.

These stories are collected and shared, with love, by Alnaaze, Louise and Tracy. We are grateful to the writers who were courageous enough to share their stories, whether endearing, funny, painful, or traumatic. Thank you all for your trust.

Let's Talk About Porn

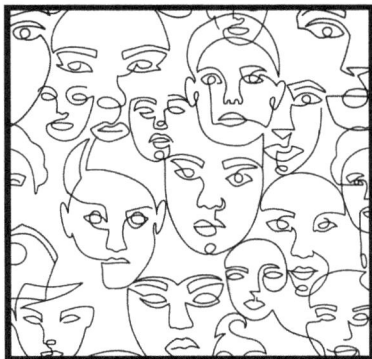

LET'S TALK ABOUT PORN

By Alnaaze Nathoo

The fact of the matter is – I love reading. Anything I can get my hands on, really. Books, magazines, whatever. I'll complain about it after if it's shit, but I'll still read it because I have this ridiculous need to understand it. And so, when I was fourteen years old and found the hidden porn stash, my habits took over. I had to read and assess everything. To this day, the fact that I spent so much time on that nonsense gives me a bit of a headache.

I don't remember exactly how I came to find the hiding place. It was this strange tiny closet-like space in the basement where we would store our suitcases. I mean, why the hell did I even go in there? It was even hidden in the wall of the insane storage place. Really, there was absolutely no reason for me to find anything at all. But, as fate would have it, I did find it, and all sorts of questions and thoughts appeared. They still haven't left me, but what I discovered may not be what you expect.

I don't actually think it was a bad thing that I found the hidden porn stash, or that I tried to understand it. Definitely not. It gave me something new to read, plus it taught me at a very early age that any crap can get published as long as there's someone out there to read it.

So it definitely wasn't this mad traumatic experience. It didn't confuse me or make me want to only have a sexual relationship with Vulcans or anything (although...). Looking back, I'd even say that it was an important part of my sexual growth and understanding. I was still at the stage where I was watching *Adventures in Babysitting* on repeat, so I was not exactly the target audience. However, I was also at an age where I understood enough about sex to know that what I was seeing didn't make a lot of sense. While I realised that it was porn and inherently sexual, and most likely there to stimulate some kind of arousal, I found it to be strange, unrealistic, and most importantly, extremely unhygienic. However, this discovery also turned out to be surprisingly educational and even liberating.

First, I discovered the magazines. For those porn aficionados out there, you'll know that to get to the articles, you had to go through a number of extremely ridiculous, highly uncomfortable, and yet eerily similar images. It seemed like every person in the magazine had to look similar to be included – which was true, of course. As I flipped through the images, the common themes, as I'm about to explore, made them very uninteresting, even for my hormonal and still maturing brain. I haven't looked at porn since, but I'm assuming that hasn't changed much. What I can say is that if consumers of porn use these images as an aid to define acceptable body types, we are all doomed.

First, every image made it clear that for a woman to be deemed as worthy for inclusion, giant breasts were a necessity. As all chesty women can attest, naturally large breasts sag to varying degrees, and generally flop to the side when one lies down. The breasts featured here were not like that. Instead, they were the kind that pointed straight up and weren't likely to move even during an earthquake, whether or not a good sports bra was involved. Depending on the situation, they could probably also shoot laser beams out of them (I'm sure this hypothesis has been tested in magazines to which I do not, thankfully, have access).

Second, every single waist was stupidly small. Seriously, none of those women had all their ribs, and that was *before* Marilyn Manson (allegedly) made that a thing. Corsets and the potential removal of some bones were definitely likely. Not to mention a diet that probably consisted of cocaine, water, and cheese. Maybe even cocaine sprinkled on cheese. Like salt.

Third, and this was the one that stuck with me the most: everyone had the same damn hairstyle – long. Some may have had bangs. I don't remember, but the hair was the usual boring colours. Mostly blond and brown, with a redhead thrown in for some diversity. They all had very long hair on their heads, and no hair anywhere else. All white people, because obviously.

Fourth, there seemed to be a standard pose: each woman had one hand opening up the vulva exposing the clitoris, and the other hand was in their mouth. Whether lying on their backs (laser boobs pointing upwards) or crouching on their knees (laser boobs pointing forwards), the set up was the same. Not particularly creative. Those poses were so unnatural, it made me wonder how those poor women could actually pose that way without bursting into laughter. Is this something that is practised at home, in front of the mirror, to get it just right? And honestly, *why* would you practise that pose in front of the mirror? Why that pose at all? So many questions!

Clearly, I wasn't the target audience because all it did was make me want to do a few stretches and make sure I was wearing a bra. I am glad I didn't spend too much time on the images, viewing them as a benchmark for female beauty and desirability, otherwise I would have been done for (though not to fear, where the images in the magazine didn't destroy my self-esteem, fashion and beauty magazines picked up the slack – but that's a story for another day).

The images were just a useless distraction, and after that quick but thorough analysis, forgotten. The important part, and also the truly confusing and educational part, was the article. As I said, I love to read. So when I realised that my discoveries had some reading in them, I had to read what was written. It would've been against my nature not to.

Another one of my fantastic quirks is that I have no problem reading the same book over and over. There are books that I have read more than a dozen times. I've read *20,000 Leagues Under the Sea* at least ten times and each of my *Nancy Drew* books were read so many times the pages were literally falling out. Every time I read one, I find that I often catch details I missed the first time and I learn something new about the characters, the setting, and some strange and wonderful detail that might not be relevant but is nonetheless absolutely exciting. I applied the same logic here. I needed to understand and therefore I read and re-read the story to see if I had missed some important plot or character point. Analysis was key to cracking this code. But is there really some kind of code in porn? Some kind of literary key?

Reading an article in a porn magazine when you're around fourteen years old, having never had any previous exposure to porn and a very limited understanding about what function porn fulfils in the overall literary landscape, is a very strange experience.

To begin with, the writing was a disaster. The plot was basic, the use of language simplistic, and the structure was messy. Too many adjectives describing the same sentiment. Kind of like a Michael Bay movie, but with a smaller budget. Admittedly, though, it was a better story. The story went something like this:

Woman loses her wallet somewhere, woman reports it stolen. The police find the wallet and a police officer comes to her home to return said wallet. They both say hello, the woman says thank you for returning my wallet. The woman and police officer then proceed to have a night of mad sex.

Much like when I saw the images, I had *so many questions*. First of all, do police really come by your house to return a stolen wallet? Or would you have to go to the police station and pick it up? Also, and really most importantly, how do you go from 'Thank you for my wallet' to 'Come in so I can suck your dick'?

As I read and re-read, trying to understand how they got from a situation of acquaintance to intimacy faster than a Ferrari, I began to move beyond what seemed to be the absolute absurdity of the situation to an interesting lesson on agency and consent. Did it seem insane to me that two random people who had barely met decided to have sex one evening? Sure. What was absolutely clear in the story, and an interesting take considering what some porn looks like even now, was that it was, however badly written, a simple story about desire, consent, and absolute acceptance.

There was no forcing or pressure and absolutely no shame. Modern societal expectations surrounding women's sexual behaviour are often very rigid and pay very little attention to how a woman experiences sex, intimacy, or desire. Women are not supposed to explore their desires or their sexuality in any way. Instead, women are supposed to look for comfort and security. Heaven forbid they actually enjoy getting laid. But not in this article with Mr Hot Policeman. The woman was happy to get back her wallet, decided she wanted a night of crazy sex with the policeman to say thanks, he was willing, and everyone was happy. It was like a few arias of feminism in what was otherwise a clearly misogynistic opera.

Surprisingly, this theme was repeated in my second discovery in this secret hiding place. I found a video tape, and much like the magazine, this was another Bay-ian Opus. To this day, I could not describe with any certainty if there was a story at all. However pointless it was, the unintentional lesson, it was an important one.

Two women, flight attendants, get off a long flight and leave the airport to catch a chauffeur-driven car to take them to what I am assuming was their hotel. After some general chit chat, one of the women pulls a long cylindrical contraption out of her bag. The object seemed to be a signal for both of the women to start masturbating. Then, while masturbating, they share the dildo as they move it back and forth between them as they pleasure themselves. They are watching each other masturbating, moving this cylindrical object back and forth in the back of their car. The driver looks in the rear-view mirror and sees this happening, and so, quite logically, he pulls out his penis while driving, and starts masturbating while watching the women in the mirror.

That's pretty much where I turned off the VCR (yes, I'm old). Even more so than with the article, I had so many questions about this scene. First of all, and something that still really bothers me: is this even hygienic? The first thing I always do after getting off a plane is take a shower and wash my hair. We all know airlines are just too cheap to clean anything properly. So why would people who actually work in airlines and know how absolutely gross they are decide to randomly share a dildo after a flight? Next, did they really have to do that in the car? How could this be comfortable? Presumably they're going to the same place – why not just wait to get to the hotel or apartment so they can get naked (and take a shower) before playtime? Third, wouldn't they just be tired after working a flight? Fourth, wouldn't that make a mess in the back seat (the hygiene again...)?

Of course, there is also the issue of driver, and that led to a whole other list of questions. Now I understand that many people drive with just one hand on the wheel. I'm guilty of that, too. But driving and masturbating? Isn't that dangerous? He'd have been much too distracted to focus on the road. Plus, in the video, he was always looking in the rear-view mirror, watching the ladies in the back pleasuring themselves. So his eyes weren't on the road at all. How did he not get into an accident? With his masturbatory driving, there is also, once again, a hygiene issue. When he ejaculates, he'll make a mess all over himself and his car. Did he have a stock of wet wipes available? Are drivers often prepared for such eventualities? *So many questions.*

Despite all of these questions and confusion, much like the magazine article, I can't say exposure to this video was 100 percent negative. First of all, I'm pretty sure it taught me how to masturbate. And while I know it's not something generally talked about, I think we can all as women admit (even if it's just secretly to ourselves) that however we learned to masturbate, it was an important lesson. It brings back the importance of pleasure in sexual experiences, including how to pleasure ourselves as well as learning to show those we choose to be intimate with how to pleasure us. A woman can and should enjoy sex, whether it's with a partner, a strange rubber device in the back of a car, or her own fingers. And despite my questions about hygiene and practicality, it was clear that the women were enjoying themselves.

While I can't say I'm a big fan of porn in general, I'm not exactly a religious purist who is anti-porn. I've always been a big believer in letting people be. The important thing here, and the lessons I drew from this exposure, were about agency, independence, and pleasure.

These stories were my first exposure to sex (outside of a sex ed 'let's look at the uterus on the overhead projector' kind of way) and provided some important lessons. While I doubt this was the point of either the article or the film, they showcased women who made choices for themselves, choosing their instincts and their pleasures. These were women who were not worried about how society would judge them based on a set of unrealistic rules and expectations created to limit and control women instead of letting them lead their sexual lives. They simply chose to lead their best sexual lives with their own rules. Perhaps I was overanalysing or extrapolated the wrong messages from the information placed in front of me, but as far as I am concerned, those are good lessons to learn.

Shame

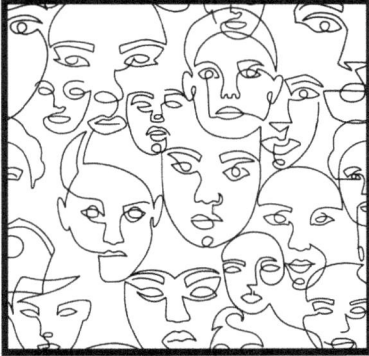

SHAME

By Aditi Banerjea

I live between two languages. On the whole, it is a blessing. But at times, I have slipped up and slipped right between the cracks. Rather than womanfully straddling the ever-shifting tectonic plates of these two languages and the cultures that they embrace, I've fallen right into the gulf that separates them.

This is one such story, or rather, it is two.

I was twenty-one and a virgin. And not entirely by choice. While my friends were falling in love and friendship with the boys who later became the men they would marry, I spent my university years almost entirely overlooked by members of the opposite sex. The one boy who professed any kind of interest in me also made it clear that it was because neither of us had done any better or indeed had any options and so, hey, why not each other? It wasn't very romantic. The one boy-man I had deep feelings for did not feel the same way about me. I wasn't devastated. Raised as I was by very traditional Indian parents, my lack of romantic options made me a very, very good daughter. Too good, in fact. Who wants to be *that* good at twenty-one?

One sultry evening in Kolkata, my mother, aunts and I sat together, stewing in the monsoon humidity. Over *shingaras* and tea, they bantered about their favourite subject: marriage. Who had married well, who had not. Who would marry well, who would not. Who was unmarriageable, who was not, and so on and so forth. The conversation rolled over comfortably.

There's something convivial about these gatherings. I might not have said much, but I was complicit. I too knew how to appraise a woman, a potential bride for the family.

The fairness of skin. Wheatish, if you please.

The slimness of gait.

The lightness of foot.

How to spot noses and lips which were in proportion.

Tall but not too tall.

Educated, preferably with a PhD, but willing to give it all up to raise children.

Charming enough to keep 'our boy' happy, but not so charming that she would steal him away and leave only room for herself in his heart.

No chronic illnesses, which included asthma.

Preferably in possession of a brother so that in her parents' dotage, the burden of responsibility should not fall on her (and by extension on 'our boy') but on that brother.

I knew the score and weddings were exciting. I had never attended one. I'd only seen them against the vast canvas of Indian films. I wanted to attend one and I was willing to offer up any woman as casual sacrifice in order to do so.

And then the conversation turned to me. My mother was very worried that no one would ever marry me. Too dark, too fat, too short, too opinionated. My aunts, being aunts, assured her that I was perfectly marriageable and that the world was my oyster. I would, they attested, have rich pickings. They just had one criteria for me: I was not to ruin myself. I was to ensure that I remained – and I translate here – unspoilt. After my wedding, they assured me, I could have all the fun I liked.

They drew closer. I was the only niece, they said, who they felt close enough to say this to. The other two were spoilt. *Noshto*.

My cousins were cool. I didn't want to be this dull, virginal block of wood that they wanted me to remain. So I jested that I too was spoilt, *noshto*. I wanted them to know that I too had been wanted, at least once. My cousins had boyfriends. I just wanted the universe to gift me the feathered touch of desirability. Even though it was a lie, I didn't want to be the ideal – this paragon of virtue. The ideal was no fun.

Pin-drop silence. No doubt my aunts were imagining me writhing around with an assortment of men, spoiling myself for my future husband. My mother hissed at me to help her bring in the *roshogollas*. She hissed at me that seeing as I didn't know Bangla very well, I should just learn to keep my mouth shut.

The word *noshto* returned to haunt me a couple of years later when I least expected it: the morning after my wedding night.

I did everything by the books. I married young. I met my

husband at twenty-three, married him at twenty-four and lost my virginity to him on my wedding night. My aunts should have been ecstatic. Incidentally, they are. I am the example that is given to every other young woman in my family. These days, to say that this sickens me and is hugely embarrassing is an understatement.

With marriage, I brought in a whole new set of aunts into the picture and, with them, I brought in a whole army of sisters-in-law.

After my husband and I met, we had a long-distance relationship. On the few occasions we met, every touch was momentous and every glance electric. Everything was heightened. To cut a long story short, we were gagging for it. Policed as we were by both our families and intent as we were to not disappoint our parents, we resisted the urge to sneak off together and rebel. We went with the flow, rebelling only during the times we were alone together, which basically meant being alone, individually, in our bedrooms, thousands and thousands of miles apart. I had phone sex before I had sex. By the time we actually got married, we had wound each other up into a state of nervous sexual frenzy.

Indian Hindu weddings take about five days and ours took slightly longer because of other assorted customs from various parents' various villages. The families effectively married each other; we were just the chess pieces that were moved around. By the time our union was socially sanctified, all the ancestors that we have ever had should have been singing from the heavens. No ritual was overlooked. It did not matter how debasing the ritual was for me as a woman, it was performed and with my blessing. I was so glad to have been chosen and loved by this beautiful man after two decades of being told that this was an impossibility that I would probably have walked over hot coals to keep my family and his happy.

Our wedding night immediately followed the wedding itself, but that night, my 35-year-old sister-in-law lay down in between us and ensured that we took turns sleeping. Apparently, it was bad luck for both the bride and the groom to sleep at the same time. Something had happened long ago and now this was a ritual. She naturally favoured her brother and his sleep over me and mine, which meant that on the night of my wedding, I was not allowed to sleep at all. She never woke him up and she didn't allow me to close my eyes.

The following night, I slept next to three sisters-in-law while my newly minted husband slept next door. There was a superstition, story, or family legend attached to every single deferral.

We grinned and bore it. My husband was used to this stuff, but I was less so. Still, I was the virginal bride and I was expected to welcome this deferral. Looking forward to my wedding night – I was told by both my husband's family and mine – was the hallmark of a spoilt girl. It was an act of *noshtami*. Good girls, the good and virtuous brides, didn't want sex; sex was just something they tolerated. Sex was shameful and to be kept under wraps. It was solely for the purpose of begetting children. Nothing more.

And finally, when the night came, when our marital bed was bedecked with flowers and hearts were made out of roses and spread out in the centre of the fresh new sheets, the women of my husband's family pulled me to one side and began to whisper in my ear. They began to tell me their tips and tricks, things that their husbands liked, things I should try to keep my husband, to bind him to the end of my sari, to my *aanchal* so that he would not stray. I was expected to perform for him. It was meant to come naturally. I wasn't to want it or have any expectations in turn but I was, for want of a better word, to *rise* to the occasion.

When they finally left us alone amidst a storm of giggles, after all the uncles ensured that the windows were bolted and pictures of me sitting on that flower-strewn bed like a little sacrificial lamb in my *benarasi* sari were taken, I burst into tears.

The desire that had blossomed between us had been entirely extinguished. It took an age to unwind me out of the sari and to find homes for the gold jewellery weighing down my ears, my neck, my arms and my wrists. It took a further age to clear the bed of flowers. We had to change the sheets because the flowers had been infested with ants.

We were suddenly not newlyweds dying to tear each other's clothes off, we were an old married couple, gently bickering over housework.

I remember falling asleep disappointed.

Waking early in the morning, we finally moved towards each other, finding each other with the touch that had eluded us for so long. I remember not bleeding and I remember reassuring my husband that I was still a virgin and checking Wikipedia with my factoids about virginity. I was terrified, even then, mid-sex, that he would reject me. As I had understood it, bigger bodies were not worthy of love and desire. My husband had made a compromise when he had chosen me and here I was, in the act of losing my virginity to him, not in an incredible amount of pain and not bleeding.

I remember him looking baffled by my insecurity. He had no idea what I had been subjected to, not just during the wedding, but for my entire life up until that point. He had seen me cry and immediately assumed that I had developed cold feet and didn't want to be there with him, in that room and on that bed.

I remember realising then that it was true that men had it all so different. I fell asleep, sore but happy. My first time had been sweet, gentle, memorable. In the end, it had been everything that I had wanted. But within this feeling of contentment, I felt confused and relieved. I was relieved that of all the indignities heaped upon me over the course of that week, at least the bed sheets would not be taken out, reviewed and inspected.

I woke up with a start. It was surely eight o'clock. My mother had told me that sleeping in on the morning after my wedding night was frowned upon: a rule, presumably, just for new brides. My husband blissfully snored beside me.

I hastily wrapped myself in a sari that I had packed for this very moment, stuck on a *bindi*, brushed my hair and emerged from the room. Within seconds, I and my unbrushed teeth were swept away in a flurry of gossip and interrogation.

What had happened last night?

How far had I gone?

Had I allowed him to have sex with me?

Had I kissed him?

To each question, my scripted answers were to shake my

head vehemently and blush furiously. No, I was a good girl. No sex for me.

My sisters-in-law sighed in relief. Sex, on a wedding night, would have indicated that I was *noshto*. They were glad that I wasn't spoilt.

My secret was safe.

Until my brother-in-law spotted my husband emerging blearily from the room hours later and accosted him as he stomped over to the bathroom (he's still not a morning person). He whooped and crowed as he bounded back to the master bedroom – my parents-in-law's room – to report that my husband's tunic was smeared with vermillion.

The vermillion that now lay thickly in the parting of my hair, marking me a married woman, had bled all over him in the night. Or maybe the morning.

My sisters-in-law tutted. Perhaps I was a little *noshto* after all.

Glossary:

Noshto: spoilt.

Shingara: a savoury snack, which is a variation of the more well-known samosa.

Bindi: the little stickers that Indian women wear on their forehead. It's placed where the third eye was once supposed to be and it is not restricted to married women alone.

Benarasi: a variety of heavy silk saris from the city of Benaras or Varanasi in India. They are synonymous with bridal wear in parts of the country.

Object of Desire

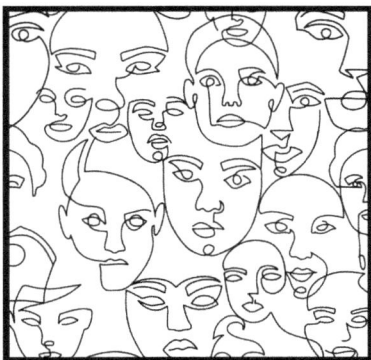

OBJECT OF DESIRE

By Jennifer Wren

I can't even remember the first time I was seen as a posses-sion rather than a whole human being with a full rich internal and external life. I do remember, though, the first time I re-alised that my sexuality would be defined by others and not by me.

When I was fourteen, I had my first kiss. Although I dressed myself up in confidence, underneath the façade I was a reserved and rather timid teenager. At a friend's birthday party, I sat on a swing seat in the garden in silence for almost an hour next to my crush before gathering the courage to reach out and hold his hand. A few weeks later, we kissed and a few weeks after that, I began hearing rumours. I heard how my boyfriend had been telling other boys about the sex we were having and how we'd been making our way through a box of condoms. Nothing I said could change the flow of gossip and nobody I turned to wanted to hear the dull truth of first base over the drama of hitting a home run.

For my high school boyfriend, his words may have merely been the result of silly teenage boy bravado and boasting. For me, his words left lasting damage, both in how others saw me and in how I saw myself. I learned that my reputation was not defined by truth and that my sexuality wasn't defined by me.

From that moment on, I became a school slut. Rumours abounded, whispers followed me in the hallways and boys suddenly took great interest in me until they realised that I didn't live up to my reputation. A lack of action didn't stop them from perpetuating the rumours, however, further branding me to boost their fictitious sexual prowess.

As I matured, so did my sexual identity, though it was somewhat crippled by my introduction to the world of sex and the damage that words as well as actions could cause. My interactions with the opposite sex, along with my consumption of media and porn, solidified my beliefs about my own sexuality: my sexual identity belonged to the world around me. My job was to fulfil those expectations, impossible as they were, as well as I could.

I convinced myself that I was in a position of power and control, ignoring the truth that I had no voice and that this identity had been moulded for me. I had not chosen it. After all, my body didn't truly belong to me.

I made my way through several unsuccessful relationships with men who had learned the art of sex through ingesting countless hours of porn. As I was contorted into one uncomfortable position after another, I would quietly feel envious of previous generations who were able to discover sex organically rather than enduring the torturous, unpleasurable gymnastics of performative fornication. If I pointed out my discomfort, they said it was my problem that I wasn't responding as I should. Time and time again, I was told what I should be doing and enjoying sexually, as men asserted that they knew my body better than I did.

It was both easy and utterly unsatisfying to be an object of desire. I was loved and wanted, I could date whomever I chose, and I received attention wherever I went, but all it gave me was a feeling of emptiness. I recall with such clarity the times I received proclamations of, 'I love you because you are beautiful!' It made my heart sink and my head filled with static. I trained myself to blankly go through the motions of relationships and engaged in perfunctory sex to please others and not myself.

When I was twenty-seven, I had a breakdown. I spent two months in a burnout clinic in Switzerland as the lone English girl who stood out amid the Swiss. Being fragile and a foreigner in a place filled with fragile people who were foreign to me made it hard to connect with others and to form much-needed companionship. Instead of friendships, the burnout clinic brought me needy, broken men.

There was Claude, the forty-two-year-old married Frenchman who worshipped me. He tried to convince his medical insurance to pay for two extra weeks at the clinic so he could spend more time with me. He hoped to leave his wife and child and start a new life together. He also added the confession that he had already had a vasectomy so I must bear that in mind if I wanted children with him in the future. He sent me unwanted pictures of his shaved naked body in the shower. I marvelled at his misplaced male confidence.

There was also Bruno, the sixty-four-year-old Austrian, who wept and told me how he loved me as he held onto my hand. Unfortunately, I struggled to understand him due to his unusually thick Austrian accent, so it took a while before it dawned on me that he was crying due to his feelings for me, rather than just being an overly emotional man.

Then there was Rüdi, the sweet eighty-year-old ex-teacher who liked to practice his English with me. Rüdi was charming and quickly became a friendly face for me at the clinic. Even at my most wary, I considered myself to be safe with an old man like Rüdi, with a loving wife at home and wobbly on his feet. One afternoon he suggested we go for a walk around the grounds. It was a pleasantly warm day for September, likely one of the last before the crisp bite of autumn took hold, so I agreed.

While enjoying a walk through the apple orchard, Rüdi asked if I would mind if he took my arm. Of course, I readily offered my arm to him, not wanting my new elderly companion to stumble on the uneven ground. A few steps on, Rüdi's grip tightened and he held me against him. I remember being shocked at his sudden strength. I couldn't escape his grasp unless I really shoved him, something I was unwilling to do to an eighty-year-old man.

Holding me close, he asked if he could kiss me. I mentally kicked myself for being so naïve as to think it was safe to be alone with an eighty-year-old. Staying friendly, I told him that I wasn't interested in a kiss and that I was just enjoying our walk. But he pressed on, repeating his request. I felt as though

I was sinking under the weight of his expectation that I would give him what he wanted, as if that was my purpose in life. I lived in a world where no didn't mean no, where I didn't belong to myself, and I was treated as an open resource for men. Finally relenting in the face of his persistence, I told him he could kiss me on the cheek – an unhappy compromise. I felt betrayed by him and betrayed by myself.

It worked, though. I grimaced as he left a sloppy mark on my cheek and then let go of me.

Back at the clinic, I told my therapist what had happened. We spoke about where I found my identity, the place my body had in my life and the lives of others, and also the responsibility I took on for others. Through the next several weeks, we worked on my boundaries and I began, for the first time, to really feel that my body wasn't a public resource or a democracy. I belonged to me. I was not a prize to be a won, an object to be worshipped, or a possession to be owned. At that point, I decided that accepting my intrinsic value was a belief worth fighting for.

The process of learning about and accepting my bodily autonomy is ongoing. I am steadily working to undo the impact of many formative sexual experiences as well as the negative influence of societal expectations that are so often placed on young women. I am thankful to have found a partner who encourages me to empower myself and to define my own sexual identity rather than allowing my value to be externally determined, whether by him or by any other means. I will no longer allow my worth as a woman to be defined by the opinions of others. Thanks to therapy, I have found my own voice and I am defining who I want to be. I know now that I am not a prize object to be owned, I don't exist to fulfil the fantasies of others, and my role in relationships is not one of subservience.

My body is mine, my sexuality is my own, and knowing this empowers me to prioritise myself and my needs, both in the bedroom and out in the world.

Feeling Flappy

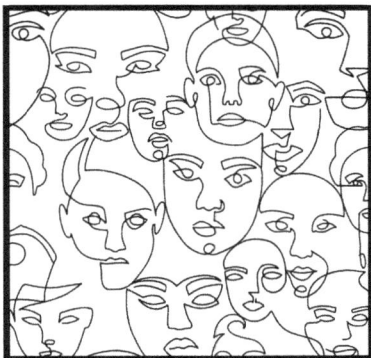

FEELING FLAPPY

By J.L. Rose

I hate my labia.

My pink taco, my piss flaps, my taffy taffy, my fleshy guardians of the love tunnel. They are the most unsexy thing about me. In my opinion, I don't have nice neat tucked-away labia. Instead, I have flaps that I can only assume resemble basset hound ears.

Let me tell you a problem with having flippy flappy labia: queefing, when you have large flappy labia, feels like it should be a hazard. What if I queef so hard I take off?

That may not really happen, but when you dislike something about yourself and are self-conscious, it's hard not to mock yourself.

They feel so gross. They don't seem normal. Everywhere around me – in books, magazines, films and porn – everyone has what is now referred to as a designer vagina. A nice neat little package that looks fabulous in and out of underwear.

Besides surgery, which I am not keen on having for something that isn't life-threatening, there isn't much I can do about them, bar tying them in a bow and tucking them away in my knickers. Maybe I am exaggerating a little, but after years of embarrassment for 'packing too much downstairs' for a woman, it's hard to learn to love them.

In sex education books and on sex education talk shows, they say, 'Everyone is different. We all have different bodies. Men. Women. Other. All different.'

Mega boobs, small boobs, lopsided boobs.

Massive dongs to micropenises.

Swing to the left, swing to the right.

Nipples in, nipples out.

Foreskin or circumcised.

Big fannies, little fannies, cardboard box.

You get my gist.

But it's still never enough for me to like what's down there. It's not commonplace to talk about our bodies with each other. Instead, we see cookie-cutter bodies while the message is rammed in our face:

This is what sexy is.

This is how you should look.

This is what people want.

It's not that anyone has ever complained or said to me, 'Cor blimey, love, what's going on with your lady curtains?' or made a fuss.

But it was always the part of me I felt most nervous about revealing when things started to heat up with someone. What if they do react? What if they say something cruel? Of course, no one ever has, so what am I worrying about?

While we're at it, I need to make sure my lady garden is bald: completely stripped back to allow more focus on my lady flower and my overgrown petals. Why must I shave off anything and everything that could signify I am a grown-ass woman? When and why did this become a necessary thing?

Some men have told me my labia are a huge turn-on. They are great, a sight for sore eyes, because it's just such a pleasure to have more to look at while they are down there. *More to look at!* Jeez, I didn't realise I could be displaying these flappy monstrosities for other people's viewing pleasure. Maybe I'm missing something here. When I pass away, maybe I should leave them to the Tate Gallery in London for others to coo at and admire.

The last thing I want, when I am trying so hard to hide or ignore something about myself during intimate moments, is for the person I am lying with or in the midst of undressing with stops and says '*Woah*, let me get a closer look! Aren't they fabulous? It's just all hanging out there, isn't it? Wow.'

Maybe they think they are doing me a favour by gushing over my baggy ham, but it makes me cringe. No matter how much I try to accept that my body is the way it is and it's ok to be made how I am, it is still a challenge.

Everyone wants to feel sexy. To look at their body and think, 'Yeah, I can see why someone would go for this.'

The rest of me is ok. Can we concentrate on those bits please? I haven't the biggest of boobs, but you get a handful on both sides. I have a bum which, I can only assume from looking at magazines and watching music videos, is in fashion now. A bum, that unlike many a celeb, I didn't have to pay for in order to have the privilege of being large and round. It's a bum that got me a lot of attention in my twenties when I hit the club. I imagine if I were twenty now, I would have the red carpet rolled out for this ass.

I'm not all about shaming myself. I do feel confident about other parts of my body. Other parts of my body do make me feel sexy.

I just get myself in a flap when it comes to my flaps.

Gargoyle Girl

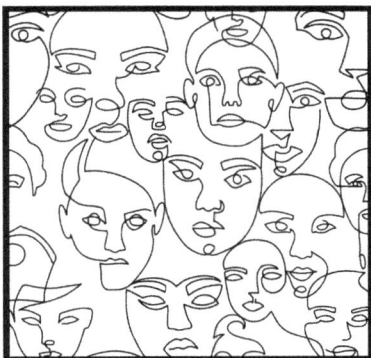

GARGOYLE GIRL

By Demona Ishimura

I remember the day my therapist asked me when I first learned about sex. In that moment, I was perplexed and unable to answer.

'Not in school with puberty class, but what I mean to ask is, when did you first understand that there was such a thing as sex?' Eleanor, my therapist, asked as she peeked over at me from behind her violet-framed cat-eye glasses. I had been seeing Eleanor for a few months. It was perhaps our seventh or eighth session together. Something about her grey high ponytail and pigeon-toed feet that didn't quite touch the ground as she sat in her tattered chintz chair was trustworthy.

'I think,' I replied, nausea erupting in the pit of my stomach and ears ringing, 'I think I always knew.'

Months prior to meeting Eleanor, I had just turned twenty-nine, graduated from college, got engaged, purchased a new home, and accepted a job related to my degree. It was an exciting time full of change and opportunity. It was as though my life had suddenly snapped together. I had been dating my fiancé for three years and was the happiest and healthiest I had ever been. In life's endless cycle, everything was swirling around and the bad inserted itself into the good. Or rather, I was finally equipped to face the bad things I had worked so hard to forget.

When this time came, I was blindsided. I went kicking and screaming to a counsellor's office for post-traumatic stress disorder (PTSD) after a series of panic attacks. I came to learn that the panic stemmed from childhood sexual trauma which I had unknowingly buried under seemingly endless memories. To this day, I am still working to piece together the broken puzzle of my youth. I have come to know her as 'Little Me' and every so often, in unpredictable ways, more about her comes up. Perhaps it is easier to separate myself from the girl who was sold for sex to men and women who were incredibly sick in the head.

It has been an interesting journey, to say the least, to move forward from this to find myself and be in a healthy spot with sex. I had a challenging time working through a lot of confusion with physical muscle memories. In retrospect, when I examine my sexual behaviour in my teenage and young adult life, there is no question that I had been abused. But I just thought that something was wrong with me. My sexual encounters before the repressed memories surfaced were awkward and forced. Subconsciously, it was ingrained in me that sex was all about pleasing the other party.

My biological parents fled the region where we had been

living when I was four years old. Lucky for me, child pornography had finally become illegal, though I didn't know that this is what drove us out of the area until much later in life. An investigation was underway and many tapes were seized from the 'copy shop' my bio mother worked for. Three leaders of the child pornography ring were arrested. The main perpetrator got six months in jail. I read his statement a few years ago when I paid to have the stenographer's notes from the hearing. He needed to provide for his two young daughters, so he got the least amount of jail time for child pornography creation and distribution.

One blustery evening, we packed up a moving truck with what we could box up quickly and drove three thousand miles away. Our pet cat meowed the whole way; she lost her voice for the rest of her life. Once we arrived at our new home town, we lived in the car and moving truck. Occasionally, I would get to be in a motel where I would earn some money. Those times are very fuzzy. I just remember tracing the outline of Donald Duck over and over again in a stencil book. The in between part is really hard. I would have taken sleeping in the car any day if sleeping in a motel meant that it would be with some abusive stranger.

About four months later, we scraped together enough money to get a house. My sister and I got to start up at elementary school again. I had my first consensual kiss when I was five and in first grade. Rami Coppe was my best elementary school friend and we played at recess every day. One afternoon, we kissed on the lips in front of the flagpole after the final bell rang. Everyone had been scuttling around to get to buses or walk home. My world momentarily slowed down when the kiss happened. I remember seeing the faintest moustache on his upper lip even then.

Eventually, Rami moved schools, then I did. We didn't make contact again until eighth grade when I learned that we had a mutual friend. This was odd considering I was so quiet that most other students in middle school thought I was mute. To make matters more confusing, I'd also met Rami Xang on the first day at my new school. Though it took a few years, I eventually developed a heavy crush on Rami Xang. For a long time, I thought that it was love.

After reconnecting, Rami Coppe and I chatted on the phone for several hours. By chatting, I mean we listened to each other breathe. We would say we'd be right back, then not actually put the phone down. but listen to the other one because we were equally ridiculous. I became highly impressed by Rami's one line of Spanish: 'Uno momento, por favor.' Eventually I agreed to attend his wrestling match.

Even from the bleachers, I could make out that moustache. There is nothing more awkward than having your first tween date be at a wrestling match. Trying to speak with someone you have a crush on when you're borderline mute is hard enough, then throw in the skin-tight uniform and nowhere to look, and it's pretty much guaranteed to be a fail. Tragically, we never spoke again. Resigned to calling it quits with my love life, my best bet was the boy down the street who I used to watch from behind our bushes as he played basketball. He'd likely never even seen me.

High school rolled around and freshman year, I plucked up the courage to ask my new crush to homecoming. His response?

'Go to hell.'

So to hell I went, and if you don't think hell is going braless to a formal dance with a group of awkward brace-face pimply outcast girls only to see the guy you asked slow dancing with what's-her-face (much cuter than you'll ever be), then you've led a nice life.

Sixteen and never been French-kissed came and went. Classmates started to pick on me and call me a prude. My closest experience to getting intimate with someone was when Travis Sharp shoved his hand down my overalls on the bus. He was in the special education classes, but his main problem was that he did drugs – a lot of them. A fifty-foot restraining order did the trick for getting him away from me.

Days before the big seventeen, I had the experience of getting kissed with tongue when Greg Prinkle followed me home from tennis practice. Red-haired and freckle-faced, he came from a highly religious family. I invited him to my room because he said he wouldn't leave until he saw it. My bio father was addicted to heroin at this point and very bad-tempered. He would be home within the hour. In an effort to make haste, I agreed to let Greg into my room which no boy had ever seen. Greg Prinkle cornered me and sucked my face off. The only thought going through my head was, 'I hate this.' What happened next was the icing on the cake, or rather the hot dog in the bun.

I don't remember what that little thing he had the audacity to whip out looked like. I simply walked out of the room when the big reveal happened. He didn't stop me from leaving. I walked all the way back to school and then walked back home. I don't know why. I guess I just needed to clear my mind. This method of resetting became a thing for me. Even to this day, if I have sex, I have to leave the room and re-enter.

When I returned home from resetting after seeing Greg Prinkle's penis, I found a red pubic hair on my comforter. I still gag at the thought of it. He works in IT now. He has six kids. I suppose that little friend of his is quite effective. Small but mighty, sheathed in red flame.

Years passed and boys came and went. By my senior year of high school, all of the flings were on the side lines and I had tunnel vision for Rami Xang. These feelings developed into college. We spent a lot of time together over nine years. We'd talk, we'd play games, we'd go to movies, hiking, on drives. I felt safe with this man. We'd kiss. We weren't just friends, but we weren't boyfriend and girlfriend because I had a boyfriend. Or two, rather, during the time I was seeing him. Rami seemed to offer something with no strings attached. The undeniable pull I felt towards him was hard for me to digest, which I think is why I dated the others.

The first serious boyfriend, whom I dated for a year, wound up being gay. I can't say I didn't know that going into the relationship. He was a good cover; I could hang out with my friends in the city where the university was located. None of those friends knew Rami. I could attend parties and lead this double life where I went back to Rami's and stopped pretending to be someone else once the parties were over.

The second serious boyfriend I had was an abusive alcoholic. I was young and dumb, so I stayed with him for the better part of a year. Hindsight is always 20/20, as they say. My perception now is that chaos was the most familiar thing from my youth, so why not carry on the tradition?

The second boyfriend was the one to take my virginity. I was nineteen. It was a mistake. We always 'did stuff' when he got drunk. It was either that or get verbally and/or physically abused. That night, he was drinking and I was sober. He took my clothes off, which caused warning bells to ring in my heart. I didn't stop it; I might have been able to.

I still wonder, though I can't dwell on this now, because did it really matter since technically I wasn't a virgin? I didn't realise it then, though. My body was doing what it had been taught to do all those years ago: comply. It was a quick in and out. I don't even know if he came. It happened in what felt like seconds. All I remember is blood and pain. He mumbled an apology about not meaning to. I stood, dressed, and walked away. Then I drove to Rami Xang's house. It was summer, it was hot out, it was late, and it started to rain. I stopped at a gas station and cleaned myself off with wet toilet paper.

When I arrived, I found Rami playing poker with some friends. He asked me what was wrong, but I shrugged it off. He shot occasional looks of concern in my direction. I joined in the game of cards. I had a few beers. Everyone left except Rami. We found our way to his bedroom. It was quiet, it was gentle, and he asked me not to leave after it happened. I left anyway. I didn't want to leave, but I left.

That was the last time I saw him. Nine years of friendship gone. They say sometimes a guy will do anything for sex. I wonder if pretending to be my friend for nine years was worth it for Rami.

I tried to call, I tried to text, and I talked to his friends, but it got me nowhere. We all want what we can't have, so I took this loss hard. He eventually got married. They had a beautiful child. Every year on his birthday, I messaged him. He messaged me back the year he got a divorce. Eventually I stopped writing on his birthday. A few times after that, he reached out and asked how I was. My replies got shorter. He finally stopped writing. I think he is happy now and possibly still single. I can't deny that I look at his shell of a social media account occasionally. There, smiling brightly, is the familiar face of the man I thought I loved for so long. Next to him is a beautiful toddler, laughter etched on her face. They're frozen in time because he never updates anything. I like to think he is too happy and busy to pop online.

I started drinking heavily after Rami left my life. I made out with anyone and everyone, and even threw in the occasional hand job for good measure. When I engaged in this behaviour, I would simply pretend like my arm wasn't attached to my body. I didn't care about what I was doing or who I was doing it with. All I wanted was to not think about him. I experienced a mixed bag of reactions to this behaviour: some men wanted to date, some became good friends, and a couple of them proposed to me.

As much as I thought about Rami, it surprises me that I haven't spoken about him until now. No one ever knew that I slept with Rami Xang. Eventually, he just became one in a number when I counted the people I've been with.

I also started to party with several different crowds so I could hear phrases like, 'Oh, you never come around,' when in truth I was drinking at least five times a week. I would get smashed and then go hide. I'd get in the back of cars and lay down and cry. I'd find a closet and slump down and wait until I sobered up. I left a drunken message on a friend's phone, screaming, 'Don't see me don't see me don't see me.' I was able to convince her I had been playing hide and seek. In truth, I would drink so much that I would flash back to my childhood. I didn't understand what was happening, so I drank more.

I would get so wasted I'd be carried off to bedrooms. I'd wake up to heavy strangers groping at me with their hot breath on my stomach or neck. I'd start to wail and cry, which most of the time scared them away. By chance, I found the boy that I used to watch from behind the hedges who played basketball down the street. One night, I hid under his bed because there wasn't anywhere better to be. He found me and calmly talked with me until I sobered up. I don't even remember what he said.

One common theme was that I hated to be sexual. It felt forced. I had guilt instilled in from me from a young age, with my biological parents frequently calling me a whore throughout my childhood. The man who was my father shamed me so much he wouldn't let me share a family bathroom. Looking back, it makes sense that he feared I was disease-riddled, considering what I was sold for as a child. Funny thing is, *that* never got brought up. He called me a slut because I talked to boys at our family business, wore shorts in PE class, and wrote a note to a boy I had a crush on. I believed for a long time that I was a whore.

Maybe that's why I kissed forty-seven people, gave hand jobs to twenty-four, and had sex with five, including the one that took my virginity. For the record, if anyone I knew had these numbers as their own, I wouldn't care because it's not me. Why is it that we always judge ourselves so harshly?

I cleaned up my act and quit drinking. I fell into a relationship with a man who'd just gotten out of prison. He was the first person I didn't cheat on with Rami, mostly because that wasn't an option anymore. This man struggled as a recovering alcoholic. I wanted to fix him, which of course was impossible, but it was a nice distraction. Spoiler alert: that whole time, I was avoiding fixing myself.

I did commit myself to him. Eventually we had sex because everyone, except for him, was telling me we should. It didn't feel right, so I went to the doctor. After a screaming panic attack in her office during a pelvic exam, she prescribed me Valium to get through sex with my boyfriend. She was the first person to diagnose me with PTSD. I ignored the diagnosis and the meaning behind it. I confided in my best friend about how horrible sex was. She gave me lots of positions to try, but I would just start to black out if I couldn't see his face, so our options were limited.

Sex was a job. My body would close down. I couldn't unclench and I'd begin to shake violently. The more I tried to suppress it, the worse the shaking became. I was always nauseated. I bled frequently. He was rather large in girth and it was quite unenjoyable. My girlfriends joked that I was lucky and they wanted a well-hung man. I do not understand the appeal.

It was the black eyes, bumps and bruises that led to us parting ways. I brought out the worst in him and it was time to move on. I was thankful to give it a rest with sex and stop pretending. My girlfriends constantly asked me what I did now that I didn't have a boyfriend. They told me I should get a dildo, but masturbation never interested me. I just didn't care about it, or my pleasure, at all.

Peer pressure led me to a store which I was told sold gargoyles, appliances, and dildos. I really do like sci-fi and gothic things, so even though my friends might have been joking, the appeal of the gargoyles was a good way to get me to a store that also sold dildos. I spent about twenty minutes learning about gargoyles from a man who, if he were painted green, would have looked like Shrek. I never saw the dildos; who knows if they were even there? I never told my friends I went. I was too embarrassed.

After that, I dated here and there, but the most serious date was one where a man told me about how he used to be obese, lost all the weight, and had to get his skin tightened. Apparently, this led to him having his nipples removed and sewn back on in a better spot. There was also allegedly some sort of surgical complication that caused him to require a catheter after this skin tightening. I'd scooted all the way to my side of the couch in the coffee shop we were at by the time he got to this part of the story. When he told me he had to avoid all magazines because they gave him painful boners, I fell off the couch. I left as fast as I could, but not before he asked if he could couch surf at my apartment for a while. After this I more or less became a born-again virgin.

One day, a song came out on the radio. I was curious about the video, so I went and watched it. In the video, one of the rapper's mannerisms reminded me so much of the basketball guy under whose bed I had hidden back in the drunk days. I couldn't stop thinking about him. It had been almost a decade since we had talked. For two weeks I went to his social media page and hovered over the 'add friend' button. Finally, one day, I did it. I pushed a button that would change my life forever.

He messaged me immediately. He said he had been thinking about me nonstop lately. I agreed to go see him and we stayed up until 4:00 a.m. talking outside of his house. He said we should elope in Las Vegas. Believe it or not, I would have done it if I didn't have a biology test the next day.

A week later, we officially started dating when he woke me up at midnight on my birthday to ask me out. Then we had sex. And we had sex again, and then again. Nonstop every day for months and months. I actually enjoyed it. As it turns out, the boy I used to watch playing basketball from behind the hedges was my best bet. We've been happily married now for three years. We still to this day have long conversations about anything and everything. I wouldn't change one minute of that.

I fell over backwards when PTSD hit, but he was there for me. We slowed down with sex because I couldn't be intimate without flashing back. He was patient then and he still is now. I don't know how I got so fortunate to find him, but the how isn't important. Some people spend their life searching for that how. What's important is that somewhere in this journey, fumbling my way through what sex shouldn't be, I found out what sex should be. I learned what sex can be. I can't succumb to any position, mind you. Our sex is quite vanilla. I still bleed every few times, which my doctor says is scar tissue. I never knew where that came from, but I guess now it makes sense.

I disowned my biological parents when they accused me of lying about the past. When I took this huge step, my life became exponentially better. This option is not the best for everyone who experiences abuse and trauma, but it was for me.

Several years ago, I heard my bio father was on his deathbed after he had a stroke, so I called him. When I announced who I was, he asked, 'What the fuck do you want?'

I told him I hope he gets better. He then told me something about the past that only I and the abuser would know. He accused me of lying about this particular thing happening. I couldn't speak. Out of shame, I hadn't told a soul about this, not even Eleanor the therapist. In that moment, whether he realised it or meant to say it, he set me free in a way. The woman who birthed me is worse than he is and I am still not able to fully capture her essence in the written word.

I still see Eleanor. She has helped me through so many things. We discuss sex a lot. Mostly it involves the past, but sometimes the only way to process these things is to face them head on, like Arwen does in *Lord of the Rings* when she faces the Nazgul. The backwards thoughts still bounce around in my brain about sex. The difference is that now I know I don't need to judge myself for them. When these thoughts arise, I turn the words into clouds and watch them sail by in my thoughts. When that doesn't work, I scribble them on paper or on my body and then go shower to reset.

I am happy to report that life goes on after abuse. Sex can be particularly troubled waters to navigate if it has a foundation in trauma. It isn't impossible to enjoy, though sometimes it might seem like it. Sex means something different for everyone and that's okay, so long as you're not abusing or exploiting someone else. There is something to be said about timing as well: I honestly feel our lives work in a way that leads us to exactly where we are supposed to be, whether that's finding that right person or learning to love yourself.

Driven to Distraction

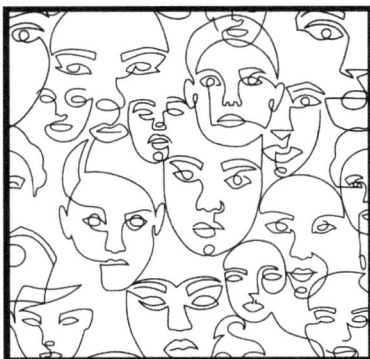

DRIVEN TO DISTRACTION

By Maggie Green

The topic of sex hasn't always been something that I found difficult to discuss. As a teen, I was quite outspoken about anything that could cause a reaction. Talking about sex worked perfectly with my peers: whether it was shock, giggles or friendly banter, it was always guaranteed to stir everyone up.

One of the people who suffered through my loud obnoxious attitude was my poor science teacher, who had been given the task to guide our class through the sex ed syllabus.

'What are condoms used for?' he asked.

The sensible students offered the answers he was looking for: 'to prevent pregnancy' and 'to protect against STIs,' but me being me, I decided that he had handled their answers far too well, so I offered my own ideas.

'Blow jobs, sir! If you don't like the taste of a penis, you can get condoms in all sorts of flavours.'

The poor guy's bald head turned a bright shade of crimson, and after acknowledging that I was technically right, he covered the answers we actually needed.

You'll be pleased to know he got his revenge a year later when I was signed up to be a youth sex educator at school. This was a project within the school where pupils were selected to be peer educators in the hope that talking about topics such as sex with kids near your own age was easier than listening to a bunch of ageing teachers. I was loud and a bit annoying, but he, along with his colleagues, thought that I would be the perfect girl to help the younger kids learn the basics of sex ed. And, not to blow my own trumpet, but I think I did a pretty darn good job. I loved standing in front of an assembly of kids, chattering away about sex, STIs, and sexual health. Nothing seemed to faze me.

Why is this relevant to who I am now? Well, funnily enough, I could talk about sex for days; it was a pretty interesting subject. But actually enjoying sex was a whole different matter.

It wasn't that I didn't like the idea, it's just that once I actually tried sex, I found it rather boring. And blow jobs... like, whoever thought they were a great idea? I'll chew on that flavoured condom minus the penis, thank you very much.

I appreciate that when you are young, you probably don't understand sex as much as you think you do. What I knew about actual sex was from gossip at school, late night dial-up browsing on the internet (followed by wiping the history clean so the parents didn't see), and Eurotrash, some weird television programme that I occasionally watched (also without anyone knowing). These were probably not the most accurate or useful tools.

Sex was painted as this glorious amazing explosive thing which happened between two people (or more, if you liked). There were scenes filled with pleasure, passion, and pain. People melted into one another as they squealed with anticipation or absolute delight. What was all this? Was this necessary? Apparently so. Since it was the only available source of information on what sex was and should be, why would it be anything else?

My family was pretty open when it came to talking about this stuff. Not that I ever really wanted to talk about sex with my family. It always felt somewhat awkward and weird.

My grandmother once offered some great advice when I tried to suggest that sex wasn't all that. She told me if I didn't fancy sex, but my partner did, I could 'Just lay back and think of England. Just get them to close the flaps once they are finished.'

As I said: awkward and weird.

And quite frankly, not what you expect your own, or any other grandma for that matter, to come out with. Soon after that, I stopped mentioning anything about sex to anyone else in case they came out with any equally peculiar suggestions encouraging me to just go for it.

I wanted to enjoy sex. I really did. As I got older, I ventured to Anne Summers, a shop in the UK that sold a whole array of sexy-time toys, clothing and accessories. I found it fascinating. I loved looking at the selection of wild and wacky things on offer, but failed to buy anything in the shop due to my own embarrassment. As I was living alone at this point, I could buy stuff online, so I took the plunge and bought myself a vibrator. If sex wasn't really cutting it, maybe I had to do something about it myself.

The vibrator came – it was one of those weird bunny ones with ears near the base to stimulate the clitoris. Now, quickly here, before I go on: *Why the heck do I want a cute bunny with erect ears to stimulate my lady parts? This is so wrong. No animal should be featured on sex toys!*

Still, I was pleased to have privately purchased this new thingamabob and subsequently put it on my bedside table for an evening of, well, we'd see. The evening came and so did I. Very briefly, I may add. A sneeze would have been the same length and had the same impact on my body. Was that really it?

Maybe, like with men, your first time experiencing real pleasure is meant to be short and sweet. Maybe with time, experience and practise, I would go on to have a long leisurely wank, or enjoy my vibrating prodding device, and be able to enjoy the full orgasmic experience it promised me. Except apparently, that wasn't to be.

Time moved on and I had a few different partners, different experiences, and different shapes and sizes. I went on to have kids and settle down. But I still wasn't finding any particular joy in sex. I could think of eleventy billion other things I would rather be doing than faffing about and making a lot of wet sticky mess. Yes, I would get excited. Yes, I would experience that sneeze-length orgasm (if you could call it that). But I would spend the rest of the time looking out the window, watching the clock or the television, wishing my partner would get on with it so we could do something else, like a nice game of Scrabble. Even foreplay was tedious. The soft stroking or caressing of my body used to tickle me uncomfortably and leave me not at all aroused.

Soon, as you can imagine, it left my partner feeling rejected and upset. Why wasn't I attracted to him? Why wouldn't I try new things? Why wouldn't I just try?

Instead, I just gave up.

I couldn't be bothered to pursue something that was so one-sided and that ultimately left me feeling used and empty. I didn't get any real joy or release with sex. The excitement faded and those sneezes of pleasure just weren't worth all the palaver.

I went to doctors, counsellors, and a gynaecologist. What's wrong with me? Why can't I just relax and enjoy sex? Why am I unable to reach a proper orgasm? Are my hormone levels ok? Am I ok downstairs? What should I be doing? Is it because I am scared of getting pregnant again?

Read this book, do this course, take this pill, get your husband to have a vasectomy. Buy more toys, try new things, be more adventurous. Try not saying no and establish a routine. Make time for sex. Regular sex will help increase your interest. Go on more dates; talk more. Try meditation, try more pelvic floor exercises. The advice kept coming. I was healthy, my lady parts inside and outside were healthy, and my hormones were normal.

Yet, something was still amiss. I couldn't change who I was no matter how hard I tried. Or sometimes, if I'm being honest, how hard I didn't try. I wasn't invested in or interested in sex. It wasn't my husband's fault. I found my partner attractive and I was in a stable home, I just got distracted and bored easily. Not just with sex, but with nearly everything.

From a young age, I'd get excited by something and throw myself into my new interest. If it didn't please me or bring me the satisfaction I was craving, I dropped it. This included hobbies, schoolwork, studying, and jobs. I needed positive reinforcement and affirmations to stay focussed. If it became a chore, I zoned out, and it was incredibly difficult to regain my interest. It was super easy for me to go from one thing to the next. I didn't really hold many things sacred, so if something was out of sight, it was out of mind too.

I was in my mid-thirties and going through my own child's diagnosis of ADHD when I was told by her therapist that I should really consider going for an assessment myself. Within the year, a psychiatrist told me I had adult ADHD. So many things started to make sense. My inability to finish or stick at things, unless they interested me or gave me immediate joy, wasn't just me being a pain in the arse. Instead, it was an actual neurological condition.

Sadly, my psychiatrist moved away and I was concerned about restarting my therapy with another person and having to recount my life story again, so I started my own deep dive into the world of adult ADHD.

Twitter became an amazing source of information. There was a huge community of people sharing their experiences along with helpful links and tools. A whole world of people like me.

One afternoon, while mindlessly scrolling through the usual gumpf on Twitter, I came across an article about ADHD and sex. Sex can affect people with ADHD differently: some craved the stimulation of sex, some were prone to taking more risks due to their impulsiveness, and others were driven to distraction (not in a good way). On a daily basis, I too was dealing with hypersensitivity to touch, carrying around exaggerated emotions after an argument or busy day, getting easily bored, and even just being zoned out of the real world. I finally felt seen.

This was normal for others, too.

So what have I done with all this newfound information? Have I sought further help? Am I now swinging from the (imaginary) chandelier? Well, no. I am a busy, normally very tired mum, with an equally tired and busy husband who works away from home. I have been through years of counselling which led to people giving me the wrong advice based on generalised sexual experiences.

Right now, I feel comfortable with who I am. Sex doesn't feature much (well, at all at the moment) in my life. For my husband's sake, maybe I should address that. I do love him, I want to be with him, cuddle him, hold him, but I just find that sex – even the thought of sex – drains me. It makes me feel resentful: why do I have to change to fit the status quo? To be whatever normal is and have a normal, healthy sexual relationship?

Maybe that's not me. Maybe it's not something I have to chase right now.

Maybe by coming to terms with who I am and embracing other worthy parts of me, things may change again. Maybe I just need to find the right help from someone who won't tell me how I need to fix my sexual desires, that my experiences are invalid, and how I should change to fit everyone else's standard of normal.

Alex's Night Out

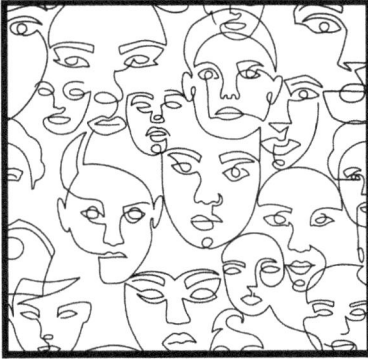

ALEX'S NIGHT OUT

By Adrian Slonaker

I stand against the wall in what is known as the gay bar. It's oldies night. On the wall is a parade of audio-visual snippets of nostalgia designed to elicit smiles and memories. It's a kind of escape, but the gay bar itself is a kind of escape from a world where I feel out of place, marginalised, or just plain fucked up. I'm supposed to be among my own kind, although even here there is a hierarchy of haves and have-nots. So I watch the grainy images of Petula Clark and Tom Jones and drag slowly on my Du Maurier cigarettes, which I know are turning my fingertips a grotty shade of gold. Yet I do it anyway because the hits of nicotine compensate for lacklustre serotonin levels. If it weren't nicotine, it would be chocolate, and too much chocolate would cause more unsightly damage than a few ochre fingertips.

I don't normally drink booze, but I want to feel something

different. I forego my Diet Coke and order an Absolut black-currant slushie. The smiling bartender, tan with muscles bulging in a way that makes me feel doughy and inadequate, cheerily hands it to me. He smiles at everyone. That's how he stays around. I suck down the sweetness, reminding me of the blackcurrant pastilles I crunched as a lonely child. But the vodka hits my head with a not unpleasant dizziness. I fellate the straw and slurp again.

I'm watching the Beatles now and also eyeing the parade of fellas marching, stumbling, sashaying past. Queens, leather men, bears, twinks, businessmen, spotty students, thoughtful types, sluts, gigglers, and the stray fag hag escorted by her loyal minions. I light another Du Maurier and yet another for the guy next to me who asks for one, flashing a flirty smile that's surrounded by thick whiskers.

'Thanks, cutie.'

I'm sharing the wealth. Building up karma, I guess. The dim smoky room reeks of liquor, sweat, and masculinity. And cologne. And desperation. I ask myself who comes here on New Year's and Christmas. Will that be my future?

I politely edge away from the drunken conversation of someone slurring incoherently. He might be trying to pick me up – or sell me drugs. Or discuss quantum physics. Thanks to his slurring and the noise levels, I can't understand him and I think I want to be left alone. Just among people, but detached. Or do I?

This other guy fascinates me. Unpretentious, blokey but not cartoonishly so, boxy-shaped, kind of like a pit bull. He seems accessible and low-key, clad in a white T-shirt (or singlet, hard to tell), leather jacket, blue jeans, and trainers. He has a receding hairline and is forty or fiftyish. It's really hard to tell, especially since I'm bad with ages.

He's sipping a beer or something like that and somewhat intently watching the Searchers performing on a *Ready Steady Go!* clip. So he likes 'Sweets For My Sweet' – so do I. On the surface, it's an innocent song for a supposedly more innocent era. He has sad dark eyes that catch my attention and nice lips that would be nice to bite. And those thick eyebrows and broad shoulders. I wonder who he is.

The Searchers end their performance to thunderous, decades-old applause on screen and the stranger turns and heads out. It's about time. It's getting late, so I follow, manoeuvring through the crowd. The air outdoors is refreshingly cool. Sweet, even in inner-city Halifax. It's springtime, the season the Dixie Cups celebrated in their achingly heteronormative (weren't nearly all of them?) smash hit 'Chapel of Love.'

I follow the guy as he takes a leafy side street. It *is* on my way home. The long way home, but still. A few blocks down, he crosses the road and stops. A few times, I think I've caught him looking over his shoulder at me and I've walked on in silence, footsteps loud and clumsy in the suspense. But now he's stopped. I stop. It feels a bit like a hunter face-to-face with a deer in a clearing. Just stopping and staring. Something has to happen.

So I get bold, maybe due to some liquid courage leftover from that vodka slushie. I cross the road towards him. He doesn't move. Soon we're face-to-face. I clear my throat and say hi. He returns the greeting and says his name is Frank.

Without fumbling, I smile and reply, 'I'm Alex. Nice meeting you.'

I've been through this routine before. I can't give my real name. I'd be too vulnerable, too raw, too flawed. If I play the part of someone else, if I channel the essence of this unknown Alex, the whole exchange will be easier and safer. I shake hands. It'd be a gentlemanly formality if I felt like a gentleman.

But I don't exactly. I don't even necessarily feel like a man. Ever since childhood, my gender identity has been like a poorly-connected electronic charger, sometimes flashing one colour, sometimes the next, sometimes not at all. Back then, one day I'd want to be Bo or Luke Duke from *The Dukes of Hazzard*, the next, Jan Brady from *The Brady Bunch*. And now? I waver between Adrian (or Alex) and Marta (or Alex), my self-perception and behaviour bobbing and flickering sometimes hourly, which can be confusing and frustrating for anyone dealing with me, least of all myself. This extends to sex, too.

Sometimes I am the raw, musky, hairy alpha beast that wants to take charge. Or I am the perfumed, obedient, tender lover fond of baby-pink silk and slow caresses. Either Adrian or Marta can be dominant or submissive, but my mind's eye views me, my anatomy and my situation differently, just as sunshine and shadows change, depending upon the hour. Sometimes I have a pussy. Sometimes I don't. Sometimes I have a dick or a large clit. I have learned to make do with what I have and a tremendous dose of creativity and willpower, which is why Adrian relished fucking a grizzled everyman's throat until he gagged and face turned lilac. It's also why

Marta let a retired soldier (whose cis-female wife waited at home) use all her orifices for his curiosity and pleasure in a bland hotel room. After shooting his load into a condom, said soldier admitted that the experience had been the strangest thing that had happened to him that year.

Right now, I am in flux. I am Adrian with Marta's eyes, which are not unlike Natalie Wood's peepers on a good day. At least 'Alex' is unisex. I peer into Frank's eyes and he studies mine. I understand. He understands. The unspoken code of queers. He asks where I live. I vaguely point towards the south.

'That way.'

He reveals that he lives on the next block and asks whether I want to stop by and hang out. After 2:00 a.m. Talk about a euphemism. I don't want to seem like too much of a whore, so I look down at my loafers and answer, 'Maybe for a little while.'

We walk on, attempting small talk. He's an accountant and part-time bartender from Toronto. It sounds reasonable. He has a vibe of urban experience and weariness, maybe even jadedness.

'I've spent time in Scarborough. I like the Bluffs.' I say it because I have to say something. I claim to be from Vancouver. 'From Burnaby,' I add with emphasis. The truth is, I did live out west for a few years when I wanted to find myself (outcome: I didn't), but I'm certainly not a native. But the Lower Mainland of British Columbia is huge and far away and 'Alex from Vancouver' seems anonymous enough but with the appropriate amount of friendliness and candour yielded by 'some name' and 'some background.' And my real life old acquaintances and relations back in Moncton won't have their conservative and religious sensitivities threatened or offended by what's about to take place.

I follow Frank inside a dull, purpose-built cluster of apartments and up a flight of stairs, then to the right, a couple of doors down. He unlocks the door and apologises that his place is a mess. Of course, it is not. Well, not much – lived in and comfortable, yes, but I don't have much time to survey my new surroundings because, as soon as my denim jacket is off, his tongue is down my throat. His meaty hands grip my shoulders (at this moment I imagine them to be like pudding, a description assigned to Inger Stevens's soft, slender shoulders on a *Twilight Zone* episode), then under my jet-black T-shirt. He comments on how furry and warm I am, and I kiss him back with equal ardour. His large mouth and pulsating breath arouse me, I'm very oral and like to kiss. I embrace him and start to massage his shoulder blades and back with sturdy fingers and velvety fingertips. He pinches my nipples hard. I gasp. Soon he pauses and clutches my fingers.

The bedroom is a bedroom, like so many others. I swiftly shed my T-shirt, jeans, socks, and shoes. He thinks it's sexy that I'm not wearing underwear. I rarely do, maybe out of laziness, but he doesn't have to know that. Let him think it's me being erotic. His body is furry, as furry as mine. A nice shape: boxy, robust, solid. It's a turn-on. I approach him and taste his mouth again, then his neck, then his chest. His cock is erect. That's a good sign. I'm doing something right. I grab my own dick-clit-dick-clit and touch it, press it, milk it as I lick his hairy flesh and inhale his armpits that give me a lift I imagine is like a cocaine high if I ever dared use that forbidden white powder. Soon I'm as hard as he is. He guides me to his king-size bed and pulls back the duvet and the top sheet. Before I know it, we are wrestling and grinding on fresh blue sheets and a duo of pillows. The body contact feels wonderful. He pins me with his legs and his arms.

He reaches over to the night table and opens the drawer. I freeze. Will he extract a knife? A gun? No. A tiny dark bottle. He unscrews the cap and brings the concoction to his nose. He inhales a whiff. I smell something heady, medicinal.

'Poppers,' he says. Then, like a perfect host, he asks, 'Want some?'

I nod, stupidly. I want the experience. Damn the consequences, whatever they may be. I mimic his snort and soon my body's senses are on overdrive, as if I were one large nerve ending. He gets on top of me and I imagine I can feel every cell of his warm flesh, every coarse hair on his body. I writhe harder, needing more of the electricity his body is conducting. He moves down me and kisses me, licks me, sucks me, and I crave more. I rub and push his semi-bald pate, his entire skull down onto my member. I want him to service me as a stud. I want the attention. All of it. But I want to suck him, too, and we contort into a 69. I need to keep the right rhythm, which is challenging, given that I'm trying to please while being pleased, despite being naturally klutzy. Soon I decide I'd rather just focus on his body, so I stop and gently nudge him back onto his pillows, tugging teasingly on his chest hair as an incentive. When he's on his back, arms behind his head, I devour his form like the wolf that I am, humping his legs before I consume his dick and balls. Then I invade his asshole with my spit-washed middle finger and thick blade of my tongue while

I continue to stimulate myself. As talented as he is, I don't trust anyone as much as my own hands.

Several times, I feel that I could climax. But I hold back, maybe for fear of missing out. He asks whether he can fuck me. He assures me that he has condoms and Astroglide. What the hell? Why not? So I pause as he grabs more supplies from the drawer. He has me suck him more to make him extra hard, sitting on my chest and lunging into my mouth. Then I hear the rip of the blue Trojan pack. He unrolls the condom – the right direction on the first try –over his dick and slathers on the lube. He applies cold drops of gel to my hole as he scans me with those sad eyes. Another whiff of amyl nitrite for him and for me. He props my legs over his shoulders. I raise my hips dutifully for the missionary position and he enters me. I briefly imagine it's Marta's first time on her wedding night.

It's quite a fine pounding, even better than I expected, as I watch his face transform into a primal, sweaty parade of expressions as he forces himself into my tightness. And the finale: he shoots his load into the condom as I drench my fist with cum. We snuggle for about five minutes, awkwardly negotiating a quasi-conversation about how we both needed that release after a busy day, as if we were two briefcase-carrying sitcom dads just back home from the office. Little does he know (or maybe he does) that I really did need it: to feel a distraction, to feel sexy, to feel desirable, to feel wanted, to not feel like an outsider with a chronically discombobulated family, to feel something akin to normal, even if I fear that my normal amounts to something hopelessly and helplessly abnormal.

I hug him again. And then I get up, using the excuse that I

have to get up early for work the next day. I get dressed, offer him a slapdash smooch on the lips and exit, proud of myself for remembering the way out and not stumbling into yet another closet in life.

My hole is sore and my face resembles a crushed beetroot from kissing and sucking. But I feel sort of satisfied. 'Sort of' because it was an empty charade of intimacy. But if we both got what we were seeking, was it really so empty? Regardless, I'd rather not focus on it.

I light another Du Maurier and perform the so-called walk of shame (although I hardly feel ashamed) to the nearest taxi rank, where at least one cabbie is usually waiting at any time. I think about the apartment-hotel where I stay, about my tiny room that, despite its shabbiness, still feels like home because it's mine and no one will criticise or judge me there. I stub my cigarette butt under my heel, slide into the taxi, sink into the seat, and sigh prettily as the meter starts. It's been a rewarding night. Sort of.

Where Pleasure
Patiently Waits

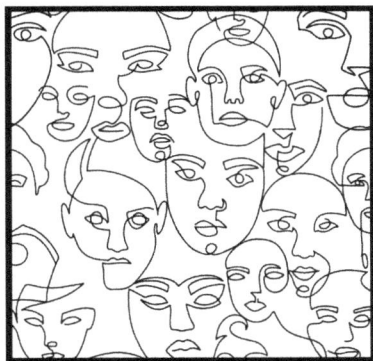

WHERE PLEASURE PATIENTLY WAITS

By Kristi Moore

What if I could tell my younger self that there would be a way to heal? What if I could sit down close beside her, look into her eyes, and help her believe there's a song she could sing to find her way out? Maybe she wouldn't have been ready to believe me. Admittedly, my suggestion would have seemed paradoxical. The very thing she thought was the enemy – her body – would be the key to becoming the lover she so desperately needed. Who could have guessed that the antidote to her troubles would be sex? And sex with herself, no less!

The thing about being able to find yourself is that you first have to admit you are lost. This is a lost-and-found love story. How could it not be? She survived, I survived, and I'm still here. This piece is dedicated to the twenty-year-old me who had no idea that sexual pleasure was waiting for her.

There have been countless attempts to make me believe

that this body of mine can only be defined by the ideals and beliefs of other people.

I am the owner of a body measured out in teaspoons and litres, tissues and stones, temperatures and cycles, conditions and symptoms, diseases and infections, minutes and years.

I am the tenant of a body filled with feelings and sensations, perseverance and trajectory, inhale and exhale, stretch and contraction, pleasure and pain, enthusiasm and regret.

Where can this owner/tenant get some distance from the close inspection of my tiniest bodily details, including the myriad of symptoms seen and unseen? How to believe them and believe myself? Where is truth hiding in this body? Is there such a thing? After all, I can almost always wonder if I was just imagining it, if I was exaggerating, or if it was something I should dismiss.

I am a collection of oddities: dandruff, varicose veins, stretch marks, pimples, wrinkles, odours, warts, hairs, plaque, stains, gas, scars, fat, mucous, blood, spit, urine, and cum, just to name a few. Seen through an emotional lens, I am an everchanging landscape of anxiety, insomnia, insecurities, dysfunction, shame, and depression. A mania leaking tears, wails, sighs, and quiet whimpers.

For every flaw, there is a cream, remedy, elixir, pill, wash, shampoo, mascara, gel, pantyliner, prick, pinch, snip, or tweeze. It's a staggering selection of products and services to ease this feeling of awkwardness-without-end. And it takes a mountain of cash (that I don't have) to buy them all.

We're taught to treat our bodies as if they are a threat. The body is a discomfiting place. Full of confusion and scepticism, it's a place to collect concerns, to be discontent, to measure up misfortunes and to wait for the next unwanted surprise. There are countless choices and sometimes none.

All inside one skin, it's a place of illogical cohabitation between hope and hopelessness. Yet this body, my body, is capable of a multitude of pleasures. And might hope and pleasure be two sides of a golden coin that was sewn into the fabric of our being at birth? After all, who taught this body about pleasure and who un/consensually untaught this body?

I have taught myself almost everything I know about pleasure. It's been a lengthy tale of trial and error. It's been a sometimes comical and sometimes tragic tale of feel/unfeel, learn/unlearn, indulge/purge, trust/doubt, grow/stagnate, forget/remember, start/stop/start again.

Again and again and *again*. In this life, I'm forever meeting *again* with a wink, a shudder, and a half-hearted (and often half-sarcastic) hurrah. It comes with a willingness to keep up the good fight whenever I can muster up my strength and courage. And believe me, there has been a lot of mustering up because I never was very good at giving up, even when I wanted to.

Again is an invitation and a chance to hope, even though hope can be a hard chance to take. Yet when I do accept the invitation and take that chance, the returns can be delicious and grand.

Sometimes it's a chance to forget what I thought about my body and the multitude of small and large disasters that can happen here. It's a chance to forget the controls and remember the sweetness of pleasure. This becomes an act of self-preservation and a protest. I can overturn their powerful hold on me and return to my Self.

There are so many ways to feel. Pleasure is just one of them – but do I dare? With all the obstacles that stand between this body and pleasure, sometimes they feel countless. Other times, the body chooses pleasure as though it were its birth right. (It is.)

In this life, birth rights seem few and far between. Most everything can be taken from me, but pleasure is a soft glowing fire in my belly that needs tending. And this flame, sometimes just a small flicker, is holding fort. It has no intention of going out and turning to ash. The fire of pleasure is patient as fuck, waiting for my yes, for the invitation to be accepted and the rightful owner of the house to take what is theirs.

If I am anything at all, I am mine. This body. My home. Yet it took me a tangled journey to be able to say: I do. I dare. I am determined.

Pleasure by pleasure, I am retelling my story by learning myself and my body anew. I am making space for a practice of tender devotion: breath, pulse, swell, surrender, orgasm. It's my very own investigation into the unknown, accompanied by curiosity for my body's nearly magical capacity to experience pleasure. It's a giving in and letting go to the expansiveness of experiences that turn my cells on vibrate and glow.

Vibrate and glow.

Vibrate and glow.

On repeat.

And with each act of pleasure, I am freeing myself from the dogma of self-loathing inspection and self-hurting repairs for a body that was never as broken as they had convinced me it was. This pleasure-seeker is not giving up and not giving in. These pleasures are mine for the taking.

Ripe and delicious and dripping sweet juices, like fruit from a tree that's no longer forbidden. It was mine all along, just waiting for me and for my willingness to say yes.

Pursuit

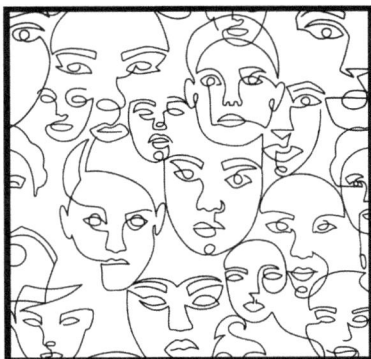

PURSUIT

By Kate Paine

Dread lodges itself like a heavy stone in your stomach the first time you think someone might be following you. It's a weight so heavy that the easiest thing in the world would be to drop to your knees even as the rest of you says *flee, flee!*

You do flee, of course, heart thrumming, feet drumming on the pavement, head swivelling as you simultaneously try to keep an eye on your follower and search for a way out of the situation and a way back into what, moments ago, was your life.

I'm fourteen, revelling in the grown-up freedom of a morning in the city with no parents in sight, darting in and out of shops, fingering the sleeves of shirts and dresses, weighing up the pros and cons of things I have no intention of buying. And there he is, staring at me from his position in front of a shop a few doors down. His gaze is hot, a heat that has nothing to do with the sweltering summer day, and everything to do with what I am, which is young, alone, and female.

I've not yet kissed or been kissed, and my notion of sex is vague, to say the least. In fact, the sum total of my knowledge comes from quizzes and articles in Dolly magazine and scenes from racy novels passed around from girl to girl at school, the relevant paragraphs highlighted in yellow or orange. Yet I know instinctively that it's my femaleness that is the lure, and that it has nothing to do with whether I've chosen the correct seasonal nail colour or learned a few choice phrases so I can communicate in the appropriate manner with boys my own age. Instead, I'm bait on a hook that, up until now, I didn't know existed.

Later, this will be a revelation that has me thinking about my mother, my aunts, my friends, their mothers, my teachers – all the females I know and don't know. I'll wrestle with the question of why no one has ever said anything and finally conclude that, if it has happened to them, then they must be embarrassed, ashamed of what their bodies can do and the effect they can have, mortified that it's beyond their power to stop it, and fearful of it happening again.

Like me, after that first time of gut-clenching fear, they'll be continually evaluating their surroundings: the light, the shadows, the footsteps behind or to the side of them, the faces of each man they pass. They'll be experts at judging in an instant the best seat to choose in a train, the best way to sit, stand, walk, run, and dance, depending on the company and the time of day. They will instinctively learn when not to draw unwanted attention to themselves and how best to go about it.

And however misguided or unfair, they will sometimes secretly suspect that they are a siren song made manifest, an inducement to touch, a magnet so strong that men intent on harming us have no choice but to act the way they do. Our culpability will be in our own hands even as theirs reach out for us.

My parents and teachers (and Dolly magazine) tell me the choice is mine: of lifestyle, sexual orientation, partner, country. I can do, or be, whatever I want, with whomever I want, where I want, and I have the strength within to make these choices and to stop others making them for me.

Hear me roar, but not too loud, because there are mixed messages, hidden undertones that seep into our consciousness, much like the whistle that only a dog hears. Be whatever you want, but be a good girl, too. Be polite, ladylike, pretty but not too pretty, forthcoming but not too much, accommodating, obliging, helpful, amenable, compliant, and indulgent.

Your body is your own, but try not to be rude.

We have no choice but to become experts in reconciling all of this, in mitigating the potentially devastating effects of the power we have on others and ourselves while trying to deal with the power they have over us.

Don't make a fuss, because what if it's all in your head?

Who do you think you are, that someone would bestow this attention on you?

What did you say to him?

Why did you wear that?

What were you thinking, staying out so late?

Did you really drink alcohol?

Were you dancing?

Why weren't you more polite when he offered to buy you a drink?

Come on, you wanted it, too, you know you did.

You hurt his feelings!

He only wanted to be friendly!

It was a compliment!

It was a joke!

You asked for it!

Get over yourself!

Here I am, fourteen and newly independent, standing on a crowded city street I've trodden many times with my mother and increasingly often with friends just like me, being watched with what certainly feels like intent by a stranger, and realising that I'm the only one who can get myself out of this situation. I'm shy, quiet, scared, and not once do I think of approaching anybody else to ask for help.

What would I say?

When I move further up the street, so does he, step for step. It's a dance, a piece of string strung between us so that when one moves, so does the other. He smiles and I quake. He gestures with one hand and I dart into a department store. It's one I've been into many times with my mother, my little brother in tow, on a mission to buy towels, shoes, a coat, a birthday card, saucepans, a piece of cake and cup of tea in the restaurant on the top floor, and to visit Santa Claus in his eyrie of fake snow in the unbearably hot Australian summer.

I run straight through to the exit on the other side and, when I glance back, there he is, walking quickly in pursuit. I run again, through the heat and my own terror, around one corner and then another, to the bus stop and onto a bus that is just leaving and which will take me home. I sit behind the driver and look neither left nor right.

I tell no one.

This is my first inkling that sex might not just be something between two people who love each other very much (thanks, Mum), or a series of fumbles in a darkened cinema or car (thanks, *Happy Days* and other sitcoms). Sex, I will come to understand, and experience, is much more complicated than that. I will eventually find out for myself that it can be wonderful, terrible, fun, messy, ridiculous, quick, slow, playful, mediocre, a panacea, an apology, a life force, a declaration of love or indifference.

Even beyond all this, it is clear that it can also have hidden depths – corners, false walls, trapdoors, tendrils that extend this way and that, ready to trip you up or hold you close. It can encompass the hot stare of a stranger, an unwelcome touch, threats, and jibes. It can have as much to do with power, fear, control, manipulation, and hurt, all of which are themes that Dolly magazine leaves well alone. It can be a weapon, powerful and devastating, leaving life, body, and mind unrecognisable. It's a fear we all learn to live with.

Over the years, it happens again in various forms: a car creeping along beside me as I stride along a city street at night, on my way to my soon-to-be father-in-law's birthday celebration; the man at the deserted suburban train station one afternoon who suddenly turns to face me with his pink penis exposed, his mouth a gaping hole of vitriol; the bar owner who tries to grab my breasts after every gig I play there and who is furious when I finally summon the courage to tell him to back off; the man who, after making a video for my band, rings me at all hours, at first cajoling but soon demanding, his language increasingly abusive and sexual, so that I ask a friend to sleep on a mattress under the window in my bedroom, just in case.

Sometimes I become fed up or infuriated and step out of this ongoing dance. I pull a bar stool out from someone who's drunk at a gig and won't leave me alone, leaning over me when I have already repeatedly told him I'm not interested. I punch someone in the shoulder when he keeps trying to take hold of the collar of my shirt and undo a button. At another gig, I tell another drunk man to fuck off when he tries to push a friend out of the way so he can grab my arm and pull me close. But even as I say or do these things, I know I have chosen moments when my safety won't really be compromised. I have assessed the risk even as the situation unfolds and my blood begins to boil. It's all second nature, this taking up the responsibility for our own safety, even as we campaign and petition, roar our discontent, march and yell and shout.

We reclaim the night again and again and again.

My daughter and I are sitting on a bench in the late afternoon sun, legs stretched out, toes wriggling in sandals that will, soon enough, be put away for the winter. That's when she tells me, hardly daring to meet my eye, that after visiting a friend in the city earlier that afternoon, she thinks she was followed on her way to the train station.

When I wrap my arms around her, her body is rigid, remnants of that urge to *flee, flee!* still lingering. I hold her tight and eventually her breathing slows, her shoulders dropping

with relief at having had the courage to say the words out loud
– more courage than I had at her age.

This is the girl who, at fourteen, still has a rotating roster of
stuffed animals by her pillow, who sings like an angel, who can
spend hours in the water until her fingers no longer resemble fingers, who has tried to teach our cat to read. This is the
girl who borrows my hats, shoes, books, socks, earrings, and
scarves, and who has now moved on to my guilt and shame
and confusion.

'I'm so sorry, sweetie,' I say and tell her it's happened to
me, too. She's a little bit shocked, I can see, because, of course,
her first instinct is to think that somehow she is at fault, that
it's because of something she has done, something that she is.
To find out that her mother has also experienced it is both a
relief and distressing, and to then find out that this is an experience she shares with nearly every woman on the planet is
simply overwhelming.

But there can be comfort in numbers and I suggest she discusses this with her friends. They'll be the next generation to
reclaim that night, to arm themselves with words and moves
that might save them or at least give themselves time to escape,
to look out for each other, to rejoice in their bodies and their
sexuality.

For kids her age, sex has a currency that was absent when I
was fourteen. It's a language they recognise even if they're not
yet fluent themselves. They learn it from school sex education,
the internet, movies, books, friends, YouTube, Snapchat, and,
in my daughter's case, from many conversations with her
mother. We've discussed men and boys, bodies, relationships,
friendships, privacy, respect, trust, what it means to be in love

(or not), and what it means to be loved (or not). We talk about good and bad intentions, what feels right to do and what feels wrong and how you might tell the difference, safety, boundaries, responsibility, consent, and culpability. These conversations become more profound as she gets older, and I find myself learning as much from her as she does from me.

But until now, we've never discussed how it feels to be followed by a man on a sunny Saturday afternoon. As a result of my silence, this incident comes out of the blue.

Our next conversation is a rite of passage for both of us.

There's only so much a teenager (and her mother) can take in one afternoon, but it's the start of what I hope will be an ongoing conversation about learning to judge the light and shade, the expression on someone's face, the distance between yourself and the next doorway. It's a tutorial on learning how to trust your gut, to not be afraid to scream and shout, use your fists, ask for help, run, do whatever it takes to remove yourself from danger.

None of this, I tell her, is a reflection on you, your body, your personality, your values and beliefs, and your capacity to love and be loved. Nor is it a reflection on your love of earrings or odd socks, your sense of humour or choice of friends, and your love of cats or *Gilmore Girls*.

That first afternoon, it feels like we have reclaimed, if not the night, then at least a little of ourselves that had been temporarily lost: mine long ago, hers only a few hours before. We sit there a while longer, arms entwined, and I long to keep her safe forever, away from prying eyes and hands, from unwelcome attention and touch. But I can't. She's going to have to learn how to negotiate her own way. Hopefully, she won't always do so alone. Sometimes with her mother, when she lets me, with friends, with a partner who will love her as much as she loves them, and with complete strangers who will step forward when she needs them, as long as she finds the courage to ask.

If I were fourteen again, what would I do differently? Would I yell and swear, frighten him off with my rage? Run towards him and knee him in the groin? Gouge out his eyes with my fingers? Laugh in his face? I would be horrified to think of my daughter doing any of these if it meant putting herself in more danger, but it's satisfying to imagine myself taking control and reclaiming my afternoon of freedom.

What I would do is tell my parents and discuss it with my friends. We'd talk like we never did about sex and power and fear and safety and our bodies and pleasure and consent, and what it might all mean.

Yes, that's what I'd do.

The Final Frontier

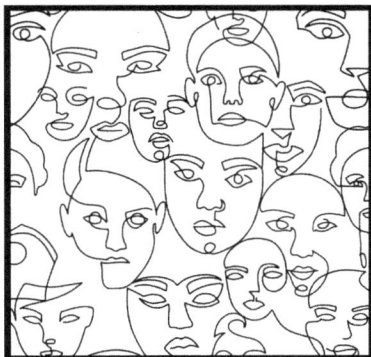

THE FINAL FRONTIER

By Jasmine James

Sex: the Final Frontier. Can you tell I'm a Trekkie? No wonder it took so long for me to lose my virginity (I was thirty).

What, in this day and age? While the answer to that is a resounding yes, it had less to do with me being a giant nerd and more to do with my religious beliefs. I live my life based on the teachings of the Bible and was brought up to believe that sex is for marriage only. My virginity was precious to me.

I'm not bothered if others hold that belief or not. It's a judgement-free zone here. For me, though, it was what I wanted. I got baptised at age eleven, which is young for someone with my faith, but I knew what I was signing up for. I wasn't forced to take my vows and I wasn't baptised at birth without my consent. I chose to take them and then chose not to break them. Even my parents were concerned that I might not fully appreciate what I was dedicating my life to, but I did then and I do now.

For the record, I am not a robot. I too have hormones and desires, even though being like Commander Data from *Next Generation* does have a certain appeal. Dude could jump high and run fast and read books and... *ok, calm down, fangirl*!

My family weren't prudes, just loving parents with a great relationship. My mum, a now-retired nurse, taught me everything age appropriate and answered all my questions. She was never visibly shocked by my questions and nothing was taboo. She told me that as long as we are open and honest about our likes and dislikes as we discover them, and we love each other, we can grow together.

I felt well prepared for if and when the time came. I dated a few men, but never felt like going further. I was always up front with them and told them at the beginning that I didn't want to have sex before marriage. They all said it was cool and they just wanted to get to know me.

It always started like that, but after the third or fourth date, they would turn to that subject. Then there were the questions, like: 'Do you think that it might happen if we really grow to like each other?' or 'Can we move forward in our relationship?'

One started off so lovely before he got pushy. I kept saying no and that he could go elsewhere, but he said it was fine. I was of two minds about whether I should stop seeing him, but we were old friends. Not that it stopped him from trying to force himself on me.

Don't worry, he couldn't walk very well for a while after

that and we didn't see each other again. I imagine he winced and walked like a cowboy for a while.

About a year later, at a London party, I met the man I eventually married. He was over from Cork, Republic of Ireland. I was won over by his big green eyes and smooth Irish voice. We were friends for a while before we started dating and it took a while before I realised I was smitten.

Once I knew, something inside me glowed like the warp core of the Enterprise. He and I share the same faith, so he got where I was coming from. It wasn't easy, as our attraction grew along with our love. Eventually, after a long-distance relationship (thank you MSN, Skype and WhatsApp), he moved and popped the question.

Our wedding day was amazing and went on till the early hours. We went to the honeymoon suite tired and happy. I was certainly disappointed when we both fell asleep. After all that waiting! How rubbish were we?

When we woke up, we boldly went where neither of us had gone before. It was natural, organic, and just like that, I wasn't a virgin anymore. It felt amazing and there were explosions of happiness.

I will admit that I was expecting a huge epiphany and literal fireworks, not just figurative. Instead, we lay there and snuggled, which made me feel loved and safe. There was no awkwardness. I think that's because we had talked frankly about sex and our relationship. I was certain when we got married, but that feeling afterwards reinforced that I had made the right decision.

I will admit that we did have to do a bit of a walk of shame as we left the hotel. We tried to sneak off without breakfast, but our families and friends had stayed there too. I was mortified when they met us with big grins on their faces.

For me, waiting till my wedding night was well worth it. Six years on, I'm still grateful for my mum's honesty and words of wisdom as I grow in life and love with my Number One (that's another Star Trek reference – I'm not hoping for another husband).

Accepting My Kinky Self

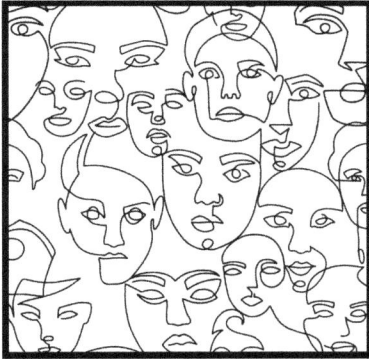

ACCEPTING MY KINKY SELF

By Yael R. Rosenstock Gonzalez

I can't remember a time before I was kinky. The first time I experienced that warm tingling feeling in my groin, I was probably six years old and watching TV. *Tom & Jerry*, *The Nanny*, *I Love Lucy* and others offered me multiple opportunities for arousal with their spanking scenes and other kink inspirations (I wonder if the networks realised). As I started high school, I switched to romance novels depicting strong-willed women submitting, after a struggle, to dominating dark and broody men who were simultaneously loving and passionate. I always loved reading, and this allowed me to imagine myself within the scenarios – the reason I prefer erotica to porn to this day, actually.

Despite my reservations about sharing what I considered a deep dark secret, my kink seemed to ooze out of me. I have no recollection of sharing my naughty desires, but my regular lovers were all aware of my spanking kink, even in my teens. My partner from my first healthy relationship was particularly good at incorporating spanking in a way that felt sexy and natural without my needing to voice anything. Spanking was an unnamed consequence when I challenged him to physically wrestle and inevitably lost. My relationship with him was the first time I felt comfortable leaning into my kinks for two reasons: he also seemed to enjoy them, and he created a safe atmosphere where I knew I was respected, loved, and valued.

After him, I found that I could get people to spank me, but it wasn't necessarily based in the power dynamics I craved. Unfortunately, I wasn't able to voice what I wanted because I failed to claim my kinkiness until my twenties. I couldn't reconcile my desire to be dominated with my ideals as a feminist.[1] I thought that by being submissive, I was feeding the patriarchy and that I should be silent instead of contributing to gender-based oppression.

There was also the fact that my first real relationship, which had a sub/Dom dynamic at times, had been abusive. While I knew that my kinkiness predated that relationship, I was afraid of ending up with someone else who mistreated me and attempted to control me for their purposes rather than my own pleasure and well-being. Unfortunately, this is not an uncommon issue in the BDSM world.

There were two pivotal moments that led to my coming out. The first was a non-kinky virtual pen pal who I had met while travelling in Argentina. We had terrible sex one night and then became good friends, chatting online frequently and even visiting one another in our home countries. He made me feel like there was nothing wrong with what I enjoyed and we started an online sexual exchange; I'd send him images of myself, which would arouse both of us, and he'd write me personal erotica. It was incredibly sexy to read stories where I was the main character while validating to have someone I knew, who didn't even engage in this behaviour, write them for me.

The second moment happened while visiting a friend while he was living in Minnesota. We met up with another friend of his, and she asked, 'How can women be submissive? It's anti-feminist.' My response was immediate and foretelling of my future in the sex education/coaching world. I confidently responded that choosing to engage in behaviour that you enjoy *is* feminism in practice, while policing women's behaviours or choices is the anti-feminist act. Feminism isn't about shaming or limiting choices, it's about expanding the available options and ensuring our agency to choose. In defending the choices of unknown women, I was finally able to accept my own.

Those experiences helped me build the confidence I needed to embrace shameless sex positivity. I joined an online kink community, attended a kink sex party, and began talking about kink during my workshops. Despite this, when it came time to publish my book, which shares my submissive and spanking kinks, I paused. Publishing my kink story pushed my comfort zone to new limits.

My book ended up being read by co-workers, my college students, family members, and even my boss. In the end, it was so worth it to share vulnerability – there is nothing wrong with who I am and what I enjoy. By sharing that, others got to learn that lesson, too.

The educator in me requires that I share that BDSM dynamics are not always healthy and can definitely be abusive. There are many people who use the idea of dominance and submission as an opportunity to intentionally manipulate and mistreat people, while others may simply not be well-versed in consent and care practices even though this community is all about the explicit communication of boundaries.

I remember I was starting to date a Domme when she sent me a video that involved gang-banging, which was intended to represent a rape scene. I stopped the video once I realised, but I saw enough to shake me. Rape scenes are not one of my kinks and can be triggering to watch due to my own experiences. I broke up with her because I couldn't trust someone to be my Domme if she would send me violent porn without warning and without first having asked about my soft and hard limits.

Also, because most of us exist in patriarchal, racist, hetero/cisnormative, ableist, etc. societies, whatever your practices, self-reflection is key to figuring out your why. Upon reflection, if you find out that you are kinky or vanilla because you were born that way or in response to trauma – cool. Being kinky or vanilla are both valid, as is the reason for your preferences being innate or a coping mechanism. However, understanding yourself more deeply can help you decide if your practices are healthy and supportive or detrimental.

As I write this, I am in a loving and supportive 24/7 Dom/sub relationship with an incredible human being who has helped me embrace my submissive side without losing myself or my values. We are equal partners who share in the upkeep of our currently shared home and have constant and clear communication. We also have rules that help me become a better version of myself, along with consequences for when I break them. My own self-reflection practice has taught me that my kinky tendencies come from how I want to see my love languages manifested.

This means that I get to be assertive, independent, badass, and submissive all at the same time. I get to choose to be taken care of by someone I trust and there is nothing wrong with that – even better, that's sexy as hell!

[1] *I recognise that feminist/ism are contentious terms due to the ways in which the feminist movements in the United States have engaged in oppressive practices against women of colour and transwomen. By using this term, I seek to both recognise that history and demand that we create a feminism that proudly and loudly represents us all.*

Grinding

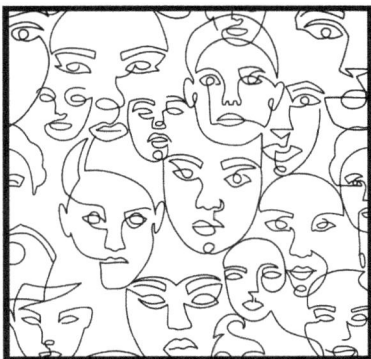

GRINDING

By Desiree-Anne Martin

It was 10:00 a.m. I pushed the button that was marked with a faded 29 and waited. The bruise around my wrist had also faded. He hated it when I was late. It made him angry and he made it known. Two days prior, he had wrapped his large, strong fingers around my bony wrist and twisted and squeezed it so hard it felt like it was in a metal vice. I hadn't cried, not only because I didn't want to show him I was weak, but also because I didn't cry anymore; there was just nothing left inside of me except a numb void. I heard the crackling over the derelict apartment block's intercom and announced my arrival. The crackling stopped, shortly followed by the click of the door unlocking.

I pushed it open with my shoulder, not wanting to touch the grimy door handle. It always made me laugh: the hypocrisy of it all. I was probably dirtier than that door handle in so many ways. The foyer was dark save for one fluorescent light that blinked on and off madly, threatening to induce seizures. I shivered involuntarily. Just a few minutes before, the sun had felt warm on my gooseflesh-covered skin as I had stood in my regular spot at the taxi rank. The foyer, in contrast, was cold, dank, and smelled of stale urine and rotting garbage. I felt bile rise up in my throat, a precursor to my episodes of projectile vomiting. I swallowed hard and rubbed my concave stomach.

Just keep it together. You're nearly there. It will be over soon.

I took the stairs to the left of the entrance, willing myself to not puke or pass out with each step. He had to live on the fucking fifth floor. And I had to be in fucking high heels.

I always made sure that I wore nice clothes and shoes and that my make-up was flawless. The make-up was mainly to hide the pitch-black circles that had found a permanent home beneath my eyes, but I had been raised to always look presentable, so I made sure I did for my job. I didn't want to look like the others. I refused to be a cliché, so, to the untrained eye, I was just another passenger waiting for a taxi at the bustling rank. Waiting for a taxi that never came. All day, every day.

I reached the fifth floor and pushed the door with my shoulder again. I felt light-headed, like the wind had been knocked out of me. I had started sweating somewhere between the third and fourth floor and wiped my forehead with the back of my wrist. I winced and gritted my teeth. I had inadvertently used my injured wrist. The pain subsided as I approached the door marked 29.

Ok, bitch. You've got this. Just keep your eye on the prize.

I knocked on the door, which opened almost immediately.

He stood in front of me, tall and muscular, eyeing me from head to toe. He seemed satisfied, his eyes shining with a mixture of lust and disdain.

'Inside.'

His accent was thick, his vocabulary limited. I did as he said and the door shut with a bang behind me, filling me with a familiar feeling of dread. I followed him to his bedroom. I wasn't sure how many people occupied that apartment, but there was evidence of several inhabitants: broken toys, piles of unwashed clothes, a stained mattress in the room we had to pass through to get to his, and a photo of him and his wife on their wedding day that was stuck to the wall above the bed with Prestick. She wasn't home. I didn't know much about him and I didn't actually give two fucks, but he had mentioned once that she worked as a hairdresser. He closed his bedroom door once we were inside and I perched myself on the corner of the bed. He had been watching porn on the small plasma TV and I hoped to hell he didn't expect me to do *that* today. I averted my eyes and looked up at him.

'How are you?'

He frowned. This was not going to be a small talk kind of day.

'Take clothes off,' he commanded. I stood up, lifted the strap of my small sling bag over my head and placed it on the already cluttered bedside table. I sat back down on the dishevelled bed and unbuckled my blue wedge-heeled shoes, then placed them neatly at the foot of the bed. He had also begun undressing, starting with his pristine white vest, then removing his expensive tracksuit bottoms, his eyes remaining on me the entire time. As I unbuttoned my nearly see-through floral short-sleeved shirt, I felt like I was swimming through syrup. I pushed my denim shorts down and placed my clothes on the office chair that occupied the one corner of the room. It was missing one wheel, so it stood lopsided, everything that had been piled on it threatening to fall to the floor. I could feel his dark brown eyes still on me as I stood in my matching underwear. That was another rule: always wear pretty, matching bra and panties. I returned to my spot on the bed, finding it increasingly more difficult to not catch glimpses of the putrid pornography on the TV.

'Do you have anything for me, baby?' I asked in my most dulcet of tones.

'After,' he replied, removing his tight boxer shorts. His already hard penis sprang up in recognition of my presence. His was large. Very large. The painful kind of large. I felt sick again. It didn't matter how many male genitals I saw, I hated them. I hated him, too, for making me wait. At least he never took very long. I bent my arms behind my back and unclipped my bra. I slid my panties off and added my black lacy underwear to the pile on the unstable chair.

'Now we fuck.'

'Yes, baby.'

I lay down on the bed, feeling entirely exposed, my small, thin naked body rigid with resistance. The pillow smelt like a woman's shampoo or body lotion, floral and sweet. I closed my eyes. I always closed my eyes. I felt the full crushing weight of his body on top of mine, followed by him prizing my legs apart with his knees. As was his want, no condom. I didn't care. There was nothing about me to care about anymore. I braced myself for the forceful penetration that was to come, twisting the sheets around both of my hands.

Chocolate. Strong coffee. The ocean. Breakfast for dinner. Massages. Long conversations with best friends. Painting. Going to the theatre. My first kiss. Shopping for clothes. An island holiday. Sunrises. Sunsets.

As he entered me with a brazen brutality, my mind frantically turned to thoughts of the things that made me feel good. Or used to, anyway. The pain surged through my fragile body and I bit my bottom lip. He kept thrusting away, groaning like the stuffed pig that he was. I tasted blood.

Just a little while and he'll be done. You're nearly there. It will be over soon.

The top of my head hit the wall hard, but he continued his repulsive rhythm, oblivious to my searing pain. History dictated that it would all be over in two more thrusts and history didn't let me down. Moaning as he came inside of me, I exhaled as he collapsed and rolled off of me. I realised I had been holding my breath throughout the entire ordeal. I inhaled deeply then immediately regretted it as all I could smell was sex. My thighs were wet with his cum and I discreetly wiped the semen off using his sheets while he lay next to me with his eyes closed. I hoped his wife would smell it later that night.

'Baby,' I whispered. 'Can I get it now please?'

He opened his eyes and looked at me, clearly irritated by the fact that I was intruding on his moment of post-coital bliss. He stretched his arm across to the bedside table and pulled the drawer open. He retrieved two crumpled R50 notes and one small teardrop-shaped piece of plastic. He handed them to me and what remained of my heart filled with the joy of a child.

Oh, sweet sweet heroin! I have waited hours for you!

I didn't ask his permission. We both knew the drill. I jumped up from the bed, grabbed my sling bag and returned to my spot. I removed my hypodermic needle, spoon and lighter and hurriedly cooked up the smack. Inserting the tip of the needle into the crook of my elbow, I shot up. I collapsed back onto the bed, this time not caring that I was fully naked, and closed my eyes, returning, as they say, to the sacred womb.

Oh, sweet baby Jesus, yes.

The sound of him putting his clothes back on and turning the volume up on the television brought me out of my glorious reverie. I walked unsteadily to the chair and got dressed. I sat on the floor and buckled the straps of my shoes. Returning all of my works into my bag, I slung it across my shoulder.

'Thanks, baby. I'll let myself out.'

He grunted, his back to me as he sat transfixed by the orgy playing out on the screen. I left his vile apartment and walked down the stairs sans the junkie withdrawal symptoms I had walked up them with. Exiting the grimy, dark building, the brilliant sunshine made me smile. I crossed the busy road and walked up the street to the taxi rank.

I was high as fuck, but the day was still in its infancy. I had to get another client for my next fix.

A Sex Toy Story

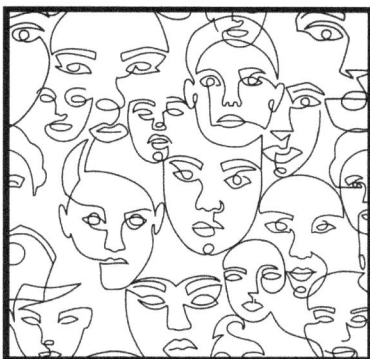

A SEX TOY STORY

By Yolanda Porter

It's one of the first muggy days of summer. Fresh out of lockdown and feeling giddy, we buy coffee in paper cups and walk to the little square overlooking the old town. In the cool shade of a linden tree we sit, keeping our distance from each other, and catch up on each other's lives. It's not uncommon in the little cosmopolitan village of Zurich to see a cluster of forty-something women from very different backgrounds sharing a joke – even if one of them is cackling louder than the rest. I'm a loud laugher; I throw my head back like I'm eating salad in a stock photo, but fuck everyone who looks at me funny for it.

There we are: three women who are happy to be out in the city, happy to be in each other's company, happy to be sharing our lives with someone we don't live with. We talk about our kids, our husbands, the work we have or have not done, and the mental space we have found ourselves in.

'I've really learned what I need and don't need in my home,' says Kate.

'I've cleaned out so much! And we haven't bought anything new the whole time,' I say, temporarily forgetting the new curtains I got installed.

Jane raises a hand. Her smile is part sheepish, part triumph.

'I've been shopping online,' she admits. She makes typing motions with her hands and in my head, I hear the joyful clacking of my husband's mechanical keyboard, which he says makes him feel productive.

'What did you buy?' I ask.

'It was bigger than I expected,' she answers, as if I know exactly what she's talking about. I don't. She waves one fist in the air, gripping something that might be an imaginary sword. 'My husband was so angry, but I love it.'

It takes the two of us a second, but for once, I catch on first. I stare at her for a moment, equating this tiny athletic woman with sex toys and only feeling bewildered.

'Why was he angry?' I ask her. 'It's not replacing him, is it?'

She laughs and shakes her head. 'We have a fine sex life. It just... it's something different. He doesn't understand why I want it, but it's – it's something extra.'

'A husband supplement,' I suggest. 'A complement to the regular stuff.'

Kate has worked it out and laughs, nodding.

'A cherry on the top!' I cry. I'm getting carried away with metaphors and innuendo now. 'The icing on the cake!'

'Anyway,' says Jane, wisely ignoring me, 'I keep it next to

the bed and now my husband gives my bedside table a filthy look when he comes into the room. He doesn't understand why I would want something like that. Like he's not good enough.'

We joke about it some more before the conversation moves on, but when I go home, I am stuck with the vision of Jane waving a fist wildly over her head, wielding her invisible weapon.

In my own twenty-odd year relationship with my husband, we have long since mapped our bodies, thoroughly established our boundaries, and explored our topography over and over, so there are no more unclimbed peaks or unswum streams. In the familiarity of the landscape is a new kind of intimacy, one that is perhaps marked by humour and comfort rather than breathless reconnaissance. Weaponised by our knowledge, we can effortlessly arouse each other with a touch in the right place, in the right way. I know the incantations that, when whispered in his ear, will weaken his knees, just as he can breathe just so in my own ear to make my stomach flutter.

It's because of this excess of intimate knowledge that we bring new weapons to bear.

This isn't to say that sex toys (even now I mentally whisper the phrase) aren't new to me. When the world wide web was just starting to become a thing, I was a frequenter of Usenet and suddenly found a vast and diverse family that wrote openly among each other about our everyday lives. With enough distance and a veneer of anonymity, tucked safely behind pseudonyms and IP addresses, we shared intimate details about our relationships, what we felt was lacking, and what we loved, hated, sought or avoided. I learned about polyamory, homosexuality, BDSM, and asexuality, all from people who lived it and wrote or spoke about it first-hand. Coming from a series of small conservative towns, none of those concepts had been more than myths and confused innuendo before. I was curious about all of them and asked questions which were willingly answered. That was when I learned about the health benefits of a good dildo.

It didn't take much convincing to get my husband into a sex shop. He was as curious as I was. My earnest attempts to seem worldly and unsurprised at the contents of a sex shop lasted until we turned into the first aisle (leatherwear, ball gags, gimp suits) and I turned to him in some combination of shock, amusement, and glee. This was a world neither of us had ever entered, and it was like entering Wonderland – if the Mad Hatter had been a Dom Queen in patent black stiletto boots.

I picked up various items and we played guessing games: what's it for? What kind of person likes that?

We left the shop with two plastic-sealed purchases in a plain paper bag and scuttled back to our car. I had the sudden guilty feeling that we would be seen by someone we knew and they would draw conclusions. The conclusions would probably be correct, too, which was the worst of it. We went home and I put the bag in our closet. Visiting the store had been such an experience, so illuminating and confusing at the same time, that I needed to process it.

We finally tested everything out one warm evening in bed: a small blue vibrator with a remote control on a cable (there was no Bluetooth in those days) and a set of vaginal beads or balls or spheres made of matching blue washable plastic.

My husband took his usual engineer's approach, asking for my subjective opinion: was A better than B, was it better like *this* (eh) or like *that* (oh!). We experimented a few times before deciding that they didn't add anything to our relationship that wasn't there already – thanks, in large part, to my analytical husband's need to try sex in every iteration and my enthusiasm.

In our decades together, we've experimented, we've gone through phases – for a while our ultimate experience was a good fuck out in nature somewhere, far from people – but without talking about it, we've settled into a rhythm that works for us both. And all we need for it is each other, a knowing hand in the right place, and the right word whispered.

We've explored our world together and wielded all the weapons we could find, and in the end, we only needed ourselves.

But if we hadn't tried them all, the intimacy and love that we create together would be something entirely different. Our openness with each other, our curiosity and fascination with *this* and *this* and what about *this*? Couldn't exist without those first times. The first time we went to a sex shop, the first time we watched porn together (laughing at the plot and trying to copy every position, often with hilarious or uncomfortable results), the first time we stopped our car on the side of a quiet road and climbed into the back seat, all created the intimacy and connection of shared experiences. Sometimes we call on the best of those first times during sex, reminding each other of our adventures. The vibrator never comes up in our recollections.

The last time I saw it was when we moved house and my mother, helping us pack, discovered it under the bed covered in dust and thoughtfully packed it in a box marked 'Very Personal Items'.

Sex toys have a valued place in any relationship that is open to them. My own experience would tell me that they can and should be part of sex and intimacy, and that trying something new and unknown, whether it works or not, adds to the shared adventure and creates new levels of intimacy and arousal. For me, personally, those are vital aspects of a strong relationship and there's nothing I would change.

Well, apart from the time we got caught naked in a cemetery, but that's a story for another day.

A Tale of a Tragic Online Dater (in 2020)

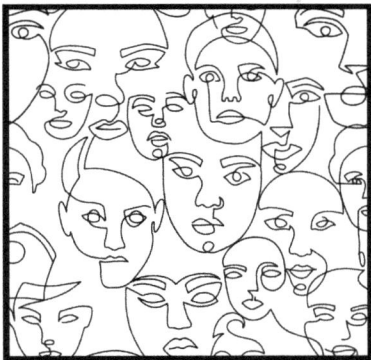

A TALE OF A TRAGIC ONLINE DATER (IN 2020)

By Carys Wiggans

Hooking up with someone in our current era is a hundred times easier than trying to find someone who will care for and love you. Just finding someone to spend your time with is harder than running a marathon with your legs taped together. You don't have to leave the house or go to a club to find someone to spend the night with, but it's practically impossible to find someone who will stick around.

I just want to go back to the days when people went on dates and the guy risked it all in trying to get a kiss – when couples went places and enjoyed each other's company. He bought her flowers and she treated him like a king.

None of that respect or romance happens today.

For one thing, pornography is so accessible and overused that it causes people to confuse the fiction of it with what a respectful partner would or should ask someone to do. In porn, women are completely objectified, always grateful, and are submissive to what the man wants. The guys watching these videos are apparently starting to think this is actually acceptable in real life.

When I started online dating, I wanted to find someone to spend time with me and who would love being together – someone who gives me butterflies.

I'm twenty-eight, I've got a good education, I think I'm a nice person, and I have a lot to offer, but that seems to mean nothing. I've never been in a serious relationship and I've never had someone tell me they love me, or even really like me. I've never been on a proper date.

With online dating, it's easy to feel like everyone else is playing a different game. I don't know how many times in the last year I've used the phrase 'I'm going to die alone' because I don't want to do what people my age expect or what I don't feel comfortable with, which leads to accusations that I'm frigid and a prude. They think I don't want sex and all I want to do is tease men and lead them on. None of this is true.

The truth is, I don't want to get my body out and send all sorts of pictures to a random person. My idea of dating is to have someone get to know me, learn about my likes and dislikes, my hobbies, my personality and my life, while I learn the same about them.

My friends always tell me that it will happen and that I'll find someone when I stop looking. That someone will be lucky and feel lucky to have me, but how long can I go on thinking I'm not yet good enough for someone?

In February, when I signed back up on the dating apps, it felt like a kick in the teeth. It was like admitting to myself that

I'm not going to be one of those girls who bumps into a guy and that's where it starts. I had to answer all sorts of questions about myself to try and attract someone. I picked my best pictures, which showed not only that I can take a nice photo, but also that I have a life and have fun.

Then came the matching process. This involved selecting the other person purely on image, which, as I am uncomfortable with my physical appearance, gives me anxiety. Not only that, but there are lads who swipe as many girls as they can to increase their chances.

At this point, the overthinking started.

Do they like the way I look?

Are they using me to have sex because they think I would put out quickly?

Did they even look at my picture?

Once there was a match, then there was the massive shock over the number of messages I received (without any previous conversation) asking for sex, telling me specific details about what they'd like to do to me sexually, or describing what they imagined me doing to them.

Apparently, it's too much to hope for a little bit of conversation first or for someone to respect me. Did they want to know my name? What I do for a living? Meet up for a date? Absolutely not. They just wanted to ejaculate on my breasts because I have a large chest.

And this is considered normal. Supposedly, this is a term of endearment these days and I should be appreciative of the compliment. Now, let's remember, I had yet to respond to these lads. I had yet to even say hello.

After matching, a few began with a good chat. Sometimes

I'd start to think, 'Hell, this one is different,' but they were just waiting until I'd given them my phone number and got off the regulated app.

As soon as this happened, the pictures of their penis were on the way. Unwanted. Never asked for. No context. Just a picture and the expectation that I'm going to jump for joy and immediately ask to meet up so I can perform all sorts of things on this wonderful penis.

The number of guys in the last six months who've sent over a picture of their erect penis? Twenty-one men.

Twenty-one idiots have sent this picture assuming this will improve their chances. Let's be honest – never in the history of mankind has a woman received a message, opened it to find a picture of a penis they didn't ask for, or want, and thought, 'Damn, I must have this in my life. This is the best start to a relationship ever.'

Instead, I end up sending the pictures to friends, asking what the hell is going on and occasionally commenting on the background, noting that they're not only exposing themselves when it's unwanted, but they're messy too.

If a man took out his penis during a conversation in real life, it would be indecent exposure, but with online dating, this is normal.

One lad talked to me for over a month. He was nice and when he asked whether we could meet up for a walk, I was excited and ready to go. However, when I asked what we would do, he told me he wanted us to go in the back of his car so I could give him oral sex.

This was also in the middle of a global pandemic and while we were on lockdown. This wasn't a one-off lad, either. They all seemed to assume meeting up for sex was acceptable. And when I say no, that not only am I not interested, but it's dangerous and I wouldn't accept even if it wasn't, then they block me.

I've asked friends for advice and their advice is:

Go with it.

You'll lose a guy's interest if you don't act the same way.

It's all a game.

Everything is so sexualised that this is considered completely normal. Rather than have a man think you're great and want to date you, he's already masturbated over you several times before you've even met. Now, I'm fully aware that there are some incredible men out there, but my experience has led to the realisation that all of this is normal now. I'm supposed to speak graphically about myself and him. I'm supposed to send pictures of intimate body parts and not think twice about it.

A couple of months ago, I'd been talking to this lad for a few days and it was going well. He asked about me, asked what I did and even managed to hold a conversation. He seemed nice and asked to go on a Skype date. I was so excited. I'd never been on a date before. I'd never had someone make it clear they'd like to explore a possible relationship.

So I got all dressed up and I did my hair and make-up. Then he called on Skype, and as soon as the video loaded, I noticed we were thinking very different things for our date. I was assuming we would get to know each other, talk about our lives, and what we want for the rest of it. He, however, had set up his camera and was sat naked on his sofa, masturbating.

When I asked why he thought this was ok, he said he liked

it when I was mad. It's safe to say I ended that call quite quickly and blocked his number.

Another time, a lad spent a whole day talking to me. There must have been over a hundred messages exchanged that day and we got to know each other. He lived near me, we had friends in common, and he seemed great. Then in the evening, he asked me to talk dirty to him. He wanted me to describe things to him so he could masturbate.

And because I said I was uncomfortable doing so, he blocked me and deleted my number. He blocked me on every social media channel we'd talked about that day.

Unfortunately, this is a common occurrence. They send a picture of them naked, I say I'm not comfortable, I get blocked. I get deleted. I get told that I would have been lucky to get them and how they were too good for me because I'm fat and ugly. They don't know what they were thinking anyway, but it was just for sex.

Now, here's the thing: I want to have sex. I just don't want to have pictures of my chubby self on other people's phones. I don't want to be with someone who's going to look at me as fat. I don't want to be self-conscious with them.

Because I know I'm chubby. I've always been uncomfortable with the way I look, but with my health conditions, it's hard for me to look how I'd like. I've never viewed myself as pretty, sexy, cute, or anything positive, but I know that on the inside, I'm great.

The thing is, with all of these apps, you don't get to meet the person. It's all about your image, how 'fuckable' you are, and how quickly you're willing to take your clothes off.

The first time I had sex, I was stuck in such deep self-hatred of my body that I got drunk and fell asleep halfway through. It was terrible, but the alcohol made me not care how I looked. It made me comfortable enough to get naked.

Sex was something I'd built up in my mind and I was afraid of being rejected for the way I look. I didn't want anyone to touch me or give them an opportunity to see me in a way I wasn't comfortable with. So I avoided it and as it built up more and more in my head, I finally just decided to go for it.

I need someone who will be understanding and will reassure me when I'm in this hatred hole. Unfortunately, I have yet to meet a lad like this.

For years, my friends laughed when they heard I wouldn't do anything sexual. I was told I was weird for being too afraid to do anything. Maybe it's not normal to build up all that pressure, but just because I'm young and don't want to have sex, I'm the one who's mocked. It's not abnormal for a woman to hate the way she looks and want to protect herself.

Now, from all of this, you're probably thinking I'm a tragic disaster, which I am, but I have had one successful story. Well, not successful, but it took longer to fail.

I matched with a lad I went to school with. He didn't know who I was, but that worked in my favour. We talked every day, all day, for two weeks. There were well over a hundred messages a day. I liked him and he was nice and respectful. He asked about my job and what I enjoy, and I hadn't seen his penis. I was thinking I was finally onto something.

And then, after two weeks of being completely absorbed with each other, he ghosted me. For anyone who's lucky enough to not know what ghosting is, it's when they read your messages and you can see they are online, but they refuse to reply. So, at this point I was wondering what I did wrong and why he no longer wanted to talk to me. What happened that it went from so good to just nothing? At what point did he decide he didn't like me and why couldn't he just tell me?

And I'll never know the answer because he'll never reply.

At this point, I've pretty much had enough of all the men who made me feel like I wasn't good enough, like I needed to be like the other girls, like I needed to show my body and enjoy rough and degrading sex.

My friends tell me I'm beautiful and amazing and guys would be lucky to have me, but all the guys I've encountered tell me differently. They tell me that I'm not enough.

Now, because of all this, I don't believe my friends and I don't listen to what they say, paying attention instead to the real opinions of the worst and trashiest men.

Perhaps I'm destined to be single. Destined to be terrible at online dating and constantly told I'm using the wrong approach and that I'm abnormal.

But if this is normal, I think I'm okay being different.

Sex and the C-Section

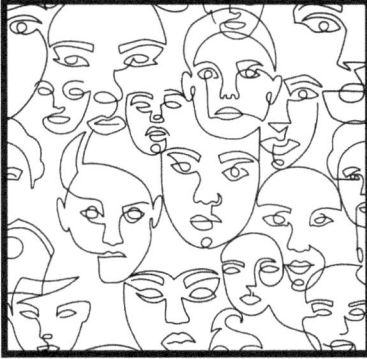

SEX AND THE C-SECTION

By L. Ferdinand

Everyone knows that after having a baby, sex is not only different, but can be quite the challenge. I knew that and didn't expect to get back on the horse any time soon, but it still surprised me how having a caesarean affected our sex life. It took probably three months before we even thought about it.

My baby was delivered by emergency C-section last summer after the baby's heart rate dropped while I was in induced labour. I hadn't really even imagined having a C-section. Instead, I'd been too busy trying to get my game face on for pushing out a baby of who knows what size.

The night before my induction, I had read up on what caesareans involved, thinking I could never be too prepared, but I didn't know if any of my friends had gotten a C-section, so I had no one to compare notes with. While I know I shouldn't compare myself to others, it would have been especially helpful regarding recovery. The pain right after the surgery was stronger than I'd anticipated. I needed morphine for a couple of days, then codeine for a few more when I was at home, and then I was down to paracetamol for a couple of weeks.

In terms of pain and discomfort, I really didn't feel normal for six months, wearing loose clothing and dresses for most of the time. Most women are aware you can't drive for a minimum of six weeks after a C-section as it's major abdominal surgery, but that didn't really bother me. I was happy to stay local and take it slowly for a couple of months. I was impressed with how quickly my wound healed, but internally, I felt like all my organs were out of place until Christmas. A friend of my mum's had a C-section more than twenty years ago and recently told me she still gets discomfort around her tummy even now, so the effects of a non-vaginal birth can last for years.

The most painful and frustrating part of post-partum sex for me was the vaginal pain. Honestly, it felt like someone was scratching nails down the inside of my vagina. It stung the whole time, making me cry out at any sort of movement. Condoms didn't help, lube wasn't a relief, and foreplay just wasn't enjoyable with the desire for enjoyable intercourse looming over us. Afterwards, I'd pee and it was really painful. The discomfort didn't last long after withdrawal, but it was very hard to experience and made for a tearful, stressful evening, which probably added to the issue.

Needless to say, the constant discomfort and pain impacted my sex life with my husband. Even a straightforward position was painful due to my sore torso. On my side, my stomach felt like all my organs were slipping sideways. I couldn't lie on my front, be lifted, or scrunch into an all-fours position.

Even while sleeping, I felt like my stomach needed to be supported, similar to late pregnancy, even though I'd fully deflated. I guess that comes with a surgeon having a rummage about in your insides. Add to that the new mum tiredness, being so busy, and being alert to a baby's cry in the next room, and sex was just not on the table (or the bed!) for a while.

For me, the frustration came from not only knowing how good sex could be, but also because I hadn't used my birth canal in delivery: no episiotomy, no forceps, nothing. There shouldn't be any damage down there, so why did it hurt so much? I knew my body had not enjoyed being pregnant, so it felt like it had decided, 'Sod this, no entry ever again!'

My husband and I did manage to communicate quite well – for once – about what was happening and he seemed to genuinely want to help. I wondered if it was a psychological thing related to post-birth trauma, so we tried lots of things to lubricate and relax. The dildo he bought me to 'help open me up a little' didn't feel much like empathy given the size and unattractive colour of the thing, but the thought was there. When things didn't go well, he understood, listened and was patient, for which I am grateful. This was my normal for a while and we worked through it.

To this day, I'm not sure what the problem was. I could blame hormones or maybe breastfeeding, which can apparently make things a little dry down there. Most likely, I think time was the best medicine. Our baby is now over a year old and things feel pretty normal again in the bedroom. I can even wear (high-waisted) jeans again, much to my delight.

My message to any reader experiencing a frustrating, painful return to normal sex after a C-section is to take your time. You've had major surgery, which it's often easy to forget. Most people have surgery in the calendar for months beforehand and can get themselves at least mentally prepared, if not physically, so an emergency intervention like this can be a curveball. Everyone recovers at different speeds and in different ways, and honestly, if I had a C-section a second time, post-partum sex would probably drop further down my to-do list. A second C-section is likely if I get pregnant again, but I imagine it will be easier since I've gone through it before and will know what to expect. We shall see.

Not Sexy

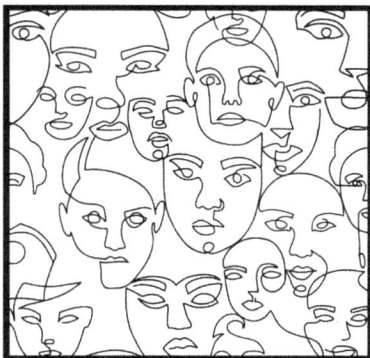

NOT SEXY

By Liam Klenk

They look deep into each other's eyes. Something clicks. They kiss. Passion overwhelms them. Frantically, they rip off each other's clothes, barely able to make it to a secluded corner. There, they fall into a tight embrace. Hands and tongues explore each other's sweaty bodies. Soon, both lovers are moaning. Their limbs become ever more intertwined, and then sweat and bodily fluids start mixing. The lovers are strong, confident, and comfortable. Their satisfaction rises in tune with their heartbeats. Their bodies are almost bursting with the need for release.

Then they climax. Together. He ejaculates. She gushes. One last powerful, muscular thrust, one last moan as the glowing lovers collapse into each other's arms.

And cut right there.

Ever since I was a child, this is what I was shown in every

movie. In every romantic scene on screen where lovers are consumed by their passion and where lust and physical satisfaction are depicted as being on an equal level with love.

This is who I felt I had to be. This is what was expected of me and what I had to aspire to. I had to be strong, in control, self-confident, sexy, driven by lust, and acrobatic in bed to be truly wanted and loved.

I tried and was found wanting.

During my attempts at one-night stands, I find myself strangely unresponsive to my lover's charms. I feel neither sexy nor excited. I am not attracted by my unknown lover's abundant suggestiveness and even caressing her feels wrong. I feel repelled, anxious, and bored, and I keep wondering how I can gently bring this to an end without being horribly rude.

In relationships, my sexual acrobatics are never up to par. No matter how much I climb around during the act, without fail, I end up making a clumsy move. Gazing romantically into her eyes, while at the same time trying to maintain the right distance between our upper bodies so I don't crush her, my whole upper body begins to shake as I try to hold the position. Sometimes a gentle fart escapes me at the wrong moment or we hold each other tight and, as we move apart, there is an air pocket between our sweaty chests, which suddenly makes a strange (and very loud) sucking noise. Nothing like this ever happens in the movies. These involuntarily comical situations often make me laugh during sex, which has irritated more than one partner.

I am not comfortable with sex. In general, I am not entirely comfortable with my body. Or rather, I am not comfortable with the role society wants me to play and what is generally expected of me.

Over the years, I have watched myself, reflected, and grew. Like most of us, I started out being rather clueless about navigating relationships in general. Now, though, as I near fifty years of age, I can say with conviction that I am a good partner. I am supportive, caring, open-minded, cuddly, warm, funny, loyal to a fault, and deeply loving.

However, lust rarely figures into my feelings for someone. I do not equate sexual attraction with love. When I fall in love with a woman, I fall in love with her mind, her eyes, and the touch of her hands. It's about the way we look at each other, support, and appreciate each other. I fall in love with her thoughts, her dreams, her potential, her passion for life, her courage, her spirit, her vividness, her vulnerability, and her kindness. I fall in love with her soul.

When I have truly fallen in love with someone, which can take months of getting to know each other, then I love kissing, snuggling, spooning, and smelling my partner's hair.

There is nothing better than binge-watching a TV series together on the couch for hours, huddling close and feeling each other's warmth. I adore the comfortable heaviness of her head on my shoulder or her legs resting on top of mine while the TV transports our minds to another world. These are moments of true happiness for me. I savour them, content with those pockets of time and wishing they would last forever.

Curling up close is great. I can't get enough of it. But every so often, while we snuggle, I will feel my partner's body language become more urgent. I will feel her tongue and hands exploring me more forcefully, which is the exact moment I find myself freezing with anxiety, not knowing what to do or how to tell her that I am not what the movies have promised.

Sex, rather than helping me in a relationship, introduces an element of stress I find hard to manage. I am not sure where this comes from, whether it's in my nature, a defect that can be repaired, a skill I need to work on, or a mental barrier I have to leap over to be free. But maybe I am free already, and the only thing amiss is the lack of acceptance for people who, like me, function differently.

I can look at my partner undress and appreciate her sexiness. In my own apprehensive way, I also want her and want to be a good lover for her. As we are not-so-intertwined, I try to do the right thing. I try to feel the passion and give her the best experience possible. Yet, after only a few minutes, without fail, my lack of sexual self-esteem triggers a spiral of thoughts. Why is this taking so long? My body is hurting. Is she happy? Am I doing ok? Damn, my arms are starting to tremble. Am I supposed to stay on top? I don't want to. I hope she is happy. Is she going to climax soon? This is taking forever.

At the same time, my body definitely reacts and trembles under her touch. I climax almost as soon as she reaches between my legs. And the feeling is explosive and glorious. Immediately after, I want to relax, fall back onto the pillows with a sigh, and cuddle for hours, smelling the enticing scent of her hair and feeling her soft skin.

I don't want to exchange too much bodily fluid. Sweat is ok, but I can't help but find discharge revolting. I almost gag when I smell or taste it. I need to fight the impulse to run to the bathroom to wash myself all over to eliminate the smell of rawness. I want to get back to breathing the tender fragrance of her skin rather than tasting our juices that erupted and flowed from deep within our bodies.

More than anything, I want to look into her eyes and see them sparkle. I can never get enough of that magical moment when she looks at me upon waking up and her entire face, her entire being, begins to light up and smile. That, right there, is true love for me. It's home.

In my experience, this makes me abnormal. Every single partner I have had possessed a strong sex drive and most of them defined love and a relationship as something which is only functional if it includes continuous, passionate sex.

I haven't encountered anyone yet who, over a longer period of time, remained satisfied with me – a loving yet sexually reserved and rather shy man who'd rather read to his partner, leaning on each other's shoulders, than take off our clothes and exchange bodily fluids.

I have tried to talk with my partners about this, but I haven't been open and honest enough. Each time, I was afraid and the words got stuck in my throat. There is a strong element of shame, impotence, and inadequacy that is attached to each of these attempts to reach out.

Also, I do not quite understand it myself. Even though I do not want much sex, I do feel sexual attraction. My body reacts to her. I can feel the butterflies when she touches me. How do I explain this as well as my reluctance to engage in sexual intercourse?

I keep trying, throughout the years, to ask for each partner's understanding and patience, hoping that together we can find a way to grow and find our own unique way of being together. But no matter how much each of my partners is in love with me in the beginning, their patience tends to run out. The rarer our sexual encounters became, the more their interest to stay loyal diminished, no matter how much we harmonised and matched in all other aspects of life.

Recently, I have had open conversations with a good number of friends and was surprised to find that some of them feel the same way I do. They, too, have to deal with the constant pressure of expectations they cannot fulfil. Their partners do not understand their reluctance towards sexual interaction either. And, they too, have spent their entire lives wondering if there might be something wrong with them.

All I know is I am more than capable of bringing happiness and love into a relationship. And in the end, isn't this what should matter most? After all, the body fades away, but loyalty and loving someone's soul does not.

I have not found my match yet. So far, talking openly about sex and finding solutions with each of my partners has turned out to be fraught with difficulty, frustration, assumptions, misunderstandings, and pain on both sides. These are conversations that are not as easy to have as I would like. In my case, the feeling of ineptitude is close to overwhelming. How can I possibly tell my partner that the more sex she wants, the more anxiety and stress it causes for me?

There's not only the stress of having to perform, and the fear of failure, but ultimately, the fear of being abandoned again.

Finding My Voice.
Period.

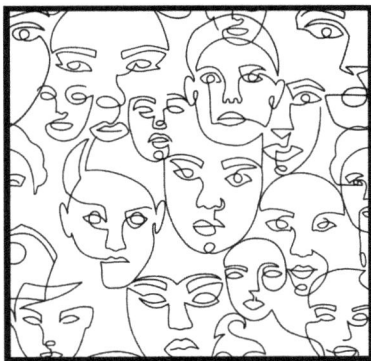

FINDING MY VOICE. PERIOD.

By Lorraine Curran-Vu

I am now a woman in my sixties, and while I have finally found my own voice, it has taken me a long time to get here. From the age of fourteen all the way into my mid-thirties, I always bought a pack of gum whenever I had to buy sanitary napkins or Tampax. I would joke to my women friends that I just needed the gum. And whenever there was a man at the cash register, I would hang around until a woman cashier became available. God forbid a guy should know I was menstruating.

I'd wonder:

Could they tell by looking at me?
Could they see through my clothes?
Could they see the outline of my pad?
Did my gait give away that I was using a tampon?

Menstruation was not only taboo for me, but also for my

women friends who were born in the fifties. The women's movement and sexual revolution took place during the sixties and seventies, but neither I nor my girlfriends felt the effects of those seminal events during our adolescence. The girls I hung around with did not talk about sex.

Attending an all girls' public school from grade seven to twelve certainly did not help me find my voice. I would wear my gym blouse to school on PE days to avoid having to show my chest to the others. And I mean chest – I did not develop breasts until I was about fifteen.

My discomfort around menstruation started, as far as I can tell, on the day my mother explained the facts of life to me. I had come in from playing with my girlfriends and was crying that they had left me out of a game.

'Things are changing, you know, Rainy,' said my mother.

'*What*?' I whined, still thinking how unfair it was that Susie chose Gail over me for her team.

Instead of comforting me, my mother said, 'Sit down, I wanna tell you something. I'll be right back.'

A few minutes later, she came back with a thin sky-blue booklet. I can't remember the title. With her back turned to me as she hulled strawberries, I was instructed to read aloud and ask my mother if I had any questions. I squirmed as I read. I looked at the black and white drawings. There was a man and a woman, fully clothed in bed. No anatomical drawings. Menstruation was explained, followed by information about sexual intercourse between a husband and wife. It was all very cut and dry.

I asked no questions. There was no mention of contraceptives and no mention of pleasure. I was glad my mother had her back to me. The whole topic made me want to finish as soon as I could so I could go outside and continue the dodge-ball game with my neighbourhood friends. I have a feeling my mother was just as relieved as I was to have the sex talk over with. Not that it was even a sex talk: I just read while Ma worked in the kitchen. Our eyes never met.

Two months later, when I was visiting my friend Susie's cottage, I saw her parents lying side by side, fully clothed, on the sofa. They were talking and relaxing.

Oh my God, I thought. *Mrs F is going to get pregnant.*

My takeaway from reading that booklet was that if a man and a woman lie next to each other, the man's sperm will jump into the woman and she becomes pregnant.

After that one booklet, my mother seemed to assume I knew all that I needed to know and that I was prepared. The only other time my mother ever brought up sex after that was when I was a college freshman and madly in love with my boyfriend.

'Don't ever come home pregnant,' warned Ma.

That was it.

That booklet had certainly not prepared me for everything. As a young teen, I was hired by my Aunt Kathy to clean her house once a week. I had five cousins in that family, three of them boys. Two of the boys were close to my age, but Tommy was three years older. Suddenly, given my new role, my cousins saw me differently: I was no longer someone they played Monopoly with or went bike riding with. Instead, I was in the servile position of cleaning up after them. I felt as if I had no choice but to suck it up since I was an eager four-teen-year-old and I wanted the pocket money.

I got a whole new perspective on them, too, as I witnessed my male cousins becoming men (and hirsute at that). The first time I cleaned the boys' bathroom, the sight of their black wiry pubic hairs in, on, and around their toilet made me want to puke. Their rooms and bathroom took me twice as long to clean as the rest of my aunt's house.

One day, while vacuuming under Tommy's bed, the nozzle started to make a strange sound and it felt as if the vacuum were sucking up paper. I scrunched down, beads of sweat forming on my brow, as I performed the Herculean task of liberating the nozzle and trying to keep my balance while investigating what was hindering me from vacuuming.

Then I saw that the nozzle was stuck on Playboy magazines, which had been strewn under the whole length of the bed. I had never seen skin magazines before. I felt paralysed. I looked into the hall, hoping that my aunt or Tommy wouldn't walk by. Had anyone seen me vacuuming under Tommy's bed? Had anyone seen me pull the magazines out?

I shut the door so no one could see me. I felt caught. My brother was the same age as Tommy, but my sisters and I were seldom allowed to enter his inner sanctuary, so I have no idea if my brother had a similar collection.

I was repulsed and embarrassed, feeling like I had done something wrong. Had I? I think back to that time, my first encounter with porn, and I hear nothing of my own voice. It felt as if I had found my cousins out and I wondered if they would somehow know. Who was at fault here? Was anyone at fault?

My older sister was the only one I told about the incident.

'Paula, something gross happened today while I was cleaning Auntie Kathy's house.'

'What?' She didn't even lift her head from her Seventeen magazine as she chewed on red liquorice.

I stammered. 'It's so embarrassing and really gross.'

'Tell me.'

'Well, when I was vacuuming Tommy's room today, I found a bunch of Playboy magazines under his bed. Tons of them.'

She dropped the fashion magazine. 'Ew, that's disgusting! You can't tell Ma.'

'I know. I feel awful. It's even hard to tell you. I feel as if I did something wrong.'

'You know you didn't. You were just doing your job. You were paid to clean Auntie Kathy's house and vacuuming is part of it, but I think you gotta keep this to yourself. Otherwise, Tommy will get into trouble and you might lose your cleaning job. Next week, just don't vacuum under the boys' beds.'

End of conversation.

I continued to clean my aunt's house for another six months. I never said a word. I never told anyone else. I continued making my cousins' beds, picking up their smelly sweaty T-shirts and musty towels, removing their hairs and urine stains from their bathroom, and vacuuming their carpet, but never under their beds.

One year later, on a Sunday morning when I was fourteen, I woke to warm sticky blood-stained sheets and underwear.

When I told my mother, she said, 'Oh, you got your period. Today's Sunday so only Hill Pharmacy is open and I don't have the car.'

Hill Pharmacy was a twenty minute walk from our house. My mother did not offer to walk there and she did not ask my older sister (who had not yet gotten her period) to go for me. Instead, Ma walked over to the sunny yellow rotary phone on the wall and made a call.

'May I speak with Tommy T., please? This is his Aunt Theresa.' She paused, then said, 'Tommy, can you do me a favour? When your shift is over, would you buy a box of Kotex and drop it off here? Thanks.'

I could not believe it. My cousin Tommy knew my secret: he knew I was having my period. My mother had just about told him. I said nothing. I did not cry. I did not ask why she had done that.

Once again, just like when I had been staring at those porn magazines under his bed, I felt like I had no voice. I had been betrayed, violated, and neglected.

Now he knew a secret about me, too. Would he look at me differently? Would he even care?

As an adult, when I think back to that Sunday when I got my first period, I am sad. My mother was in denial of my maturity. And I was too. How did I spend that morning and afternoon, waiting for Tommy to come by after his shift? I was alone in my room for eight hours, laying silently in my bed. I thought that if I were supine, I could stem the menstrual flow. I was immobilised, trying to keep life at bay, trying to stem the tides of change. I spoke to no one.

I was without a voice. My menstrual flow was joined by flowing tears because of my mother's neglect, tears that she was in denial, and tears that I myself had suppressed my own voice.

Now here I am in my sixties and I wish I had a daughter to whom I could tell this story. I wish I had a daughter to share my story of humiliation, from finding my cousin's porn magazines and thinking I was at fault to lying silently in that bed. I wish I had a daughter to encourage her to find her own voice. Although I have no children, I can still make my story heard. I can use my voice. Period.

Gospel

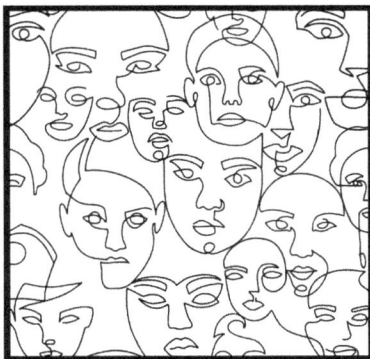

GOSPEL

By Julio Jacinto

I had a gut feeling that freshman year would be the greatest year of my high school life. This was the year that I, the lone rookie of the Taekwondo Tigers, would dominate the most prestigious and most awaited competition in the country, the Palarong Pambansa.

Or so I thought.

It all began after an intense training session when all of the boys were in the shower room. The entire place reeked of sweat and body odour and I had to cover my nose as I squeezed through bodies and slid into a cubicle. I dried my hair with a towel as I waited for the sound of slippers and chatter to subside before deciding to go outside to change. I didn't usually like changing with the team since they would yank the towel away and slap your buttocks as you curled into a ball while the others recorded the entire thing. Or at least that's what happened to my friend when he was a freshman.

To my surprise, I wasn't the last one in the comfort room. That was odd because, of all the people left, Kuya Ernie was there. He was busy fixing the chains of the silver crucifix that draped around his neck.

Kuya Ernie was a senior and apparently one of the only seniors without an attitude problem towards the younger members. As Coach's right-hand man and the most responsible black belter on the varsity team, he would usually take charge of practice whenever Coach wasn't around. He was very approachable, so I would always go to him during partner stretching and we would usually pair up in sparring sessions. He would console me after practice whenever I got berated by Coach's sermons and I would end up feeling much better after my favourite coffee drink and a few laughs. He was the older brother I never had.

Everyone knew that Kuya Ernie was a working student, so he was always the first one to take a shower, change clothes, and leave. It became a taekwondo team tradition to reserve the first shower cubicle for him. It was unusual for him to stay this late, so I asked why he was still there.

'Sorry, Ico, I was actually waiting for you,' he said. 'It was my payday yesterday and I thought I might treat my favourite freshie to dinner at Roxas.'

I found it weird for him to wait for me, knowing that he had more important stuff to do. Nonetheless, I agreed. I grabbed my bag and changed into my post-practice clothes, ready for dinner at the Roxas Night Market.

As I went for the door, his hand intercepted mine. He

pressed his back against the door and loomed over me. I narrowed my eyes and tried to reach for the doorknob again only to get swatted away once more. His mouth curved into a smirk. He slowly clicked the knob and the sound echoed across the silent room. I started to tremble.

'Is there something wrong, *kuya*?' I finally had the nerve to squeak.

I thought, at that moment, he would burst into laughter and say that this was all a joke to scare me, but he didn't. Instead, he put his hand on my head and slowly, very slowly, twirled his finger around my hair.

'*Tanggalin mo*, Ico,' he whispered as his hand made its way to the side of my face.

Those three words wrapped around my neck, slowly tiptoeing their way into my ears. I could have sworn I misheard him.

Before I could even react, his other hand started making its way inside my shirt, tracing the edges of my body. His smirk widened as his hand pressed against my chest, where he felt my heart beat so fast that I thought it would burst. I was frozen solid. He inched closer to me, head tilted until his mouth was next to my ear. What he whispered next drained the life out of me.

'Ico, *patikim lang*. Just this once. I won't tell anyone.'

I felt like screaming. I felt like crying. I felt like melting right then and there.

I felt everything at once, but I did not move an inch.

All I did was close my eyes as the tremor of fear consumed me. The next thing I knew, his hand moved away from my chest and started making its way lower, pressing his fingers on my trembling skin. The room was quiet, but I could hear my heart beat as loud as his breathing, his hands dancing to its rhythm. A frenzy of emotions coursed through my veins as I held my breath.

I felt the heat of his body against mine as he leaned toward me and closed the gap between our lips. The feeling lingered, but the thought of it stung every part of my body. He grabbed the hem of my shirt. The entire thing felt like a joke, but neither of us were laughing.

I still could not believe what was happening until he lifted me up with one swift scoop of his arms and dropped me on the sink, then glared at me like I was prey. I shut my eyes and bit my bottom lip so hard that I could taste my own blood as he started to unzip my pants. He took a deep breath and slowly sunk his fingers into my denims, pulling it to my knees. Tears started to race down my cheeks, and as I took deep, heavy breaths, he bit the garter of my boxers, pulling it down with clenched teeth. My eyes were shut so tight that they stung, but it was better than seeing the morbid image of him thrusting his head on my crotch while his warm mouth made choking sounds, sloshing with saliva that dripped on my legs. The sounds that echoed across the empty room could not be unheard.

It took an immense amount of courage to move my quivering hand. I reached for his head and managed to grasp a handful of hair. His eyes locked onto mine, then he slowly nodded at me, beckoning me to inch closer to his face again. Finally, I mustered up the courage to shut him up.

With every ounce of strength I had, I shoved him away. The tremendous force made him stumble and he groaned as his head bounced on the floor from the impact. I took this opportunity to pounce at the door, throw the door open, then run for my life.

A week later, Kuya Ernie had quit the tae kwon do team. He never told anyone why, not even our coach, but I could hear murmurs from my teammates that he decided to study somewhere abroad. I was so traumatised by the experience that I had to stop training for a month. I failed to make it to the regional finals, which was supposed to be my ticket to the national games, but I couldn't care less. Nothing was the same after that incident. I wasn't the rookie who was hungry to win, the rookie who wanted to dominate every game, the rookie everyone idolised. My dreams were utterly shattered, along with my innocence.

It was, by far, the worst plot twist of my entire high school life. It was a burden I had to carry, and I could not unload this extra baggage or open up to anyone. It was a secret that stayed locked up in a box, with the key buried at the bottom of my consciousness.

The scene kept replaying in my dreams for an entire week, which would always leave me shivering in bed, drenched in sweat in the middle of the night. I peered over the side of my bed and recalled the coldness of the silver cross that Kuya Ernie wore, the one that caressed my warm legs and spread his drool all over my skin. Then I remembered the feeling of his rough hands cradling my shivering legs, the burning sensation as he started licking my hard nipples while stroking my saliva-covered dick, and the softness of my whispers, begging him to stop.

It was like we were in church, and he was on his knees, worshipping the gospel that dangled between my thighs.

Finding the Balance

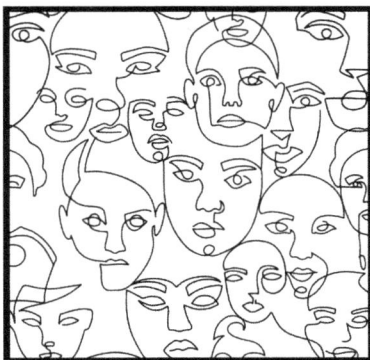

FINDING THE BALANCE

By Harmony Hurford

Sex and money are tangible routes to power. I'd even say, as these are the concepts we hold in the highest regard, that they are our reasons for being. After all, you can have and hold them both, and the more you have, the 'better' you are.

My family was never moneyed. As a child, it didn't bother me much, but that changed as I hit adolescence. My teenage years were a torrid navigation of hormonal tides, a need for my peers' approval, and a general sense of unworthiness. The transition from primary to secondary school meant new friends and new opportunities for social gatherings, including shopping, cinema trips, and sleepovers. This all comes at a price that my family could not afford. When I was fifteen, my parents divorced, and our financial struggles moved us from London to the Midlands. It was a shocking decision and I was torn from my very best friends.

Eventually, the dust started to settle on our new lives. After a rocky few months, my mum was back on her feet and, at my new school, I did end up making a new best friend. Sometimes my new best friend and I would go out drinking at the weekends in the park. This is a rite of passage for teens in the UK, especially if your hometown is stifling and wants to trap you, as smaller places tend to do.

One Friday, we were drinking with some of her friends I didn't know yet. One of them was a boy with dark hair and a sense of humour I hadn't encountered before. We exchanged details and went on a date the following week. He invited me back after and we had sex. I remember warmth and a red blush spreading across the white sheets of his bed. The pain was brief and anticlimactic.

Having sex is proclaimed as the loss of innocence or birth of womanhood in much the same way the period is and historically, both periods and sex have cast women as dirty. Periods have been noted as physically dirty, but sex is different. If a woman enjoys sex, she lacks the necessary qualities of the wife: subservience and pliability. A woman is a woman when she starts menstruating and can have children, but she isn't supposed to enjoy sex. She plays a passive role in this act. To have agency in the performance of pleasure or creating the children she also bears would be granting her too much power.

This is, of course, archaic ideology. But as a fifteen-year-old girl living in a perennial state of unrest, I was nothing but a product of the society I'd been flung into. I wasn't yet querying my awareness of the world's systems or power structures. I was given validation by a boy I thought was funny before cognisance of my trauma. I went back again and again for physical intimacy at the time I felt most alone and it felt like love.

He was busy a lot. He was a college student in the year above me and played football semi-professionally. I found the extra year between us a mark of sophistication. It was alluring for its protective implications. This is popularly termed daddy issues, though that trope in itself is wildly problematic.

He was busy, so we only saw each other on Sundays. I walked the thirty minute trek from my house to his every week in blind ritual, and we had sex for hours on end before his dad dropped me home. I'd wind up in my own bed, spent and aching, delaying my shower for as long as possible to keep his scent on my skin. For the week after, I'd sit in classes at school and cross my legs to feel that familiar twinge between my thighs. Because our relationship lacked appellation, I clung to the aftermath of our physicality. This was the tenderness where his hips met my legs. This was the memory of him cumming inside of me.

I thought about him, and our sex, all the time. The little dopamine I experienced came only from his incoming messages. I forgot about everything else. My schoolwork suffered and my friends started to call me out for my moodiness and random bouts of tears.

I'm in love, I'd say, and I can't help it.

In truth, I'd carried my family struggles with me into my teenage years and was squashing the memory of them by any means necessary. At that point in my life, I'd have picked anyone willing to give me attention.

The relationship died before it bore an official title, and I sunk into life as an entirely single teen, post-virginity. I was eighteen and consumed by the heaviness that comes from an unfulfilling relationship. I didn't have respect for myself because I defined my worth by the sexual attention I received and the only person I'd slept with had treated me as disposable. Of course, this isn't atypical. It unfortunately happens all the time. But when you're eighteen and you've been wrapped up in someone for three years, you forget this.

I started sleeping with more men. I'd form tenuous connections with them through text, sleep with them a couple of times, and then never speak to them again. I managed this well. The more sex I had, the more insouciant I became towards the act. It was entirely casual for me. I liked hook up culture and I was good at it.

Part of this haze meant I was totally unprepared for university, the next stage of my life. My parents were absolute in my going to university. But at eighteen, I wasn't ready. I felt pushed around and so took a gap year to try and regain some agency in my life.

I found a job waitressing at a little gastropub in a village just outside my city. I worked fifty hour weeks and didn't have time for much else. I became friends with the regulars, learned the pub inside out, and built friendships with my colleagues.

The front of house team were all girls. The owners had an informal policy to only hire young attractive women. I started getting very close to one of the girls who worked full time like me and we'd often do lunch shifts together in the week. She was gorgeous, of course, but I always found women gorgeous. As a child, I'd have intense friendships with one girl at a time until an inevitable argument caused the peremptory end of the relationship. These girls were always very pretty and we were touchy-feely with each other in the way eight-year-olds are. We hugged a lot, shared beds at sleepovers, or held hands when walking. This was normal to me.

The friend I worked with was different. At work we shared details of our lives to curb the general dullness of our job, as people do. She was particularly interested in my relationship status.

I'm single, I said. She didn't mention her state of affairs.

I didn't drive at this point and lived a couple of miles away from the pub. This meant I needed lifts there and back. She picked up on this and started to drive me home sometimes. Whenever I offered her petrol money, she'd say no.

One evening, she pulled up outside my house and was quiet for a couple of minutes. I was quiet, too. Ordinarily I'd say goodbye and leave the car, but something felt different.

She kissed me. I kissed her back and then left the car abruptly. I went into my house and cried in my room for two hours. At three in the morning, I texted her, saying: I'm straight.

She didn't reply. We worked together for the next week in near silence until she drove me home that Friday night. It was December and cold even in her car. My breath was coming out in silvery puffs.

We kissed again and then touched each other. She was light and delicate in my mouth, like a finely made macaron. The experience transcended my other sexual encounters. Somewhere, in the back of my heterocentric brain, I thought *this isn't even proper sex*. I was conditioned into believing that sex was a man inserting himself in a woman, dominating her and expelling within her. My fumbling in the car with my colleague was many things, but it was not this.

I didn't feel dominated, either. We were equal. In the back of her car, half naked and panting, we were dancing around each other. This confused me.

When we were finished and dressed again, I told her what I'd texted her the night we first kissed.

I'm straight, I said.

Okay, she said.

We kept having sex. In an effort to quell the effect she was having on me, I started sleeping with other men, too. We'd usually have sex in the back of her car after work, and then after, I'd text a random boy and sleep with him. As soon as his penis slid inside me, I felt better again. This was strange, because sex with my colleague was far more pleasurable than with any man. I told myself I simply hadn't found the right man and so kept finding more to sleep with.

I knew I was growing attached to her. I cut things off with us by telling her I'd been sleeping with countless men on the side.

She didn't cry. We carried on working together until I left for New Zealand in March. I came back to England to start university in September and I didn't see her again.

I'm twenty-three now. I didn't sleep with any women at university, though I know my attraction is more than simple admiration. I had a string of unsuccessful relationships with men, treating each more badly than their predecessor, but I didn't do it deliberately. I was just sad.

I didn't come out as bisexual until after I graduated. University is an institution, after all, and institutions carry the set norms society puts in place. Though I don't think anyone would've been bothered that I'm not straight, I'd always been inclined to suppress this part of myself.

When I came out, nothing particularly happened. There was the odd titillation from straight men, including talks of threesomes and the like. Now I tell them firmly that my sexuality isn't a smorgasbord for them to wash down their throat as an hors d'oeuvre. Not all sexuality caters for the straight man, despite what they may think.

In the interest of repairing my relationship with sex and my sexuality, I've been celibate for a year. The polarity of my sexual experiences with men and women isn't what I want in a partnership. With men, I've always worked to subdue. With women, it is the opposite, as though I am unleashing my pent-up sense of grief and trauma through an act that is only supposed to be love and exploration of one another.

So, until I find someone to bring that moderation out of me, I will abstain from sex. Practising celibacy has been the source of happiness I didn't think I'd find again.

The Accidental
Advocate

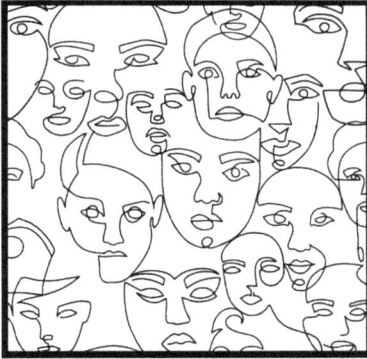

THE ACCIDENTAL ADVOCATE

By Ximena Escobar de Nogales

Another massage session with Li Hua is over. I feel relaxed, oxygenated, content. I've been coming here for years now. Her name means *pear blossom*. This fine middle-aged woman has a firm touch; her hands offer the right pressure. There is always such empathy in her touch, such care and generosity.

'*Ça va Camille?*' She interrupts my reverie, asking me about my eldest daughter, adding, '*Tulour pa copa?*'

Li Hua arrived in Geneva, Switzerland close to ten years ago, but her French is still hard to decipher. There are plenty of French phonemes that the Chinese language doesn't have and, I presume, vice versa. I always struggle to understand her.

'Camille is fine,' I say as I get up from the massage bed. 'She visited recently when the airports reopened in the UK.'

'*Til Londo?*'

'Yes, she is still living and working in London. She's been there for five years now.'

'*Tulour pa copa*?' She repeats the question. I replay the sounds in my head in an effort to make sense of them. Then I realise she said *toujours pas de copain*. She is asking if Camille still has no boyfriend.

I hesitate a second, then another.

'No, Li Hua, actually... Camille has a girlfriend,' I say. And, to make sure she understands, I add, 'Camille likes women.'

Always that brief silence, that searching for cues in the interlocutor's eyes. Did you understand what I just said? Has my revelation landed in a safe place? Are we good? Li Hua is wearing a mask covering her mouth and nose, but I see in her eyes that she is shocked. Her face looks like a surprised emoji.

'*Vous acet ça*?' She asks whether I accept *that*. She takes a step back as she speaks. And, before I even attempt to answer, she says, '*Emmen la doteul.*' Take her to the doctor.

I am stunned. This woman does not censor herself; she doesn't need thought bubbles over her head. It's all out there. That, I suppose, is good. Other people silence their disapproval.

'Camille is not sick,' I respond firmly, but calmly. I am not angry. Rather, I am disappointed and sad. We are in Geneva in the twenty-firstcentury, yet Li Hua is a product of Maoist Chinese upbringing. She was raised thinking people attracted to the same sex should be corrected and healed. I tell myself that Li Hua doesn't know any better. Later, I learn that homosexuality has been legal in China since 1997 and was declassified as a mental illness in 2001. But I am aware that even the modern open-minded liberal Swiss society in which I live breeds and harbours homophobes.

'*Et son papa?*' she asks about Camille's father.

'What about her father?' I ask, putting my dress on. For a second, as the fabric passes my head, I surprise myself by sticking my tongue out at her.

'*Il acet ça?*' She asks whether my husband accepts *that*. Then she repeats, '*Emmen la doteul.*' Take her to the doctor.

I reply, firmer this time, 'My daughter is not sick, Li Hua. There is no reason to take her to the doctor. She is a healthy adult woman: beautiful, clever, independent. I stand by her.'

'*Voulez te?*' She offers me a cup of tea, but there is something hasty in her tone and a busyness in her movements, which is new.

'No, Li Hua, not today.' I realise I, too, want this conversation over.

A moment later, I am sitting in the car with the motor off, wondering if I will ever come back for a massage.

'There is no reason not to come back,' my inner voice tells me. 'You have to be tolerant to those whose opinions oppose yours. Show them their prejudices, but be firm.'

Then another voice says, 'Don't ever come back here! This woman just denied your daughter the right to exist as she is. Tolerating that is not standing up for your daughter.' And just then, I realise I had never before been on the receiving end of a direct homophobic comment.

I drive home thinking of how many times my daughter must have experienced disapproval and rejection for her sexual orientation. I recall how discreet she always is about her girlfriends in public. And I think of how I could have responded to Li Hua with an easy answer, like, 'No, Camille still doesn't have a boyfriend.' That would have been a truthful statement and would have avoided further discussion.

But then, perhaps without noticing, don't I choose these opportunities to sensitise people about same-sex relationships? It is ignorance that must be combatted. People are afraid of the unknown. Let them meet a lesbian woman – see her face, give her a massage even, see how normal she is – and this will help break down the prejudices.

I think back to the time when I learned Camille is a lesbian. She was a teenager, eighteen maybe. If there were earlier signs, I completely missed them. She had recently been inviting a girlfriend over and I sensed this was not just another friend from school. One day I asked her,

'M isn't *just* a friend, right, Camille? Are you... in love with her?'

She gave me a warm, shy smile. Her eyes affirmed and I understood. That night I remember asking my husband, 'So what do we think about having a homosexual daughter?'

'Well, aren't we liberal?' he said, but it didn't sound like a question.

A rational, open-minded, liberal and generous man, he felt there was little to discuss. Nothing much had changed for him, except, he said, that he now knew his daughter better. The fact is, we didn't have a problem accepting Camille's homosexuality. Not having to come to terms with it allowed me to move onto the next thing: making sure others accepted her sexuality. With my mother, sisters, mother-in-law and friends, I felt an urge to inform, have them accept it, and move on.

I don't care about the gender of Camille's partner. It's

character that matters and I want Camille – and all my children for that matter – to have good, reliable, honest life partners. But I know this immediate acceptance doesn't come easily to all. I wish I could help those who struggle to accept their child's homosexuality.

On several occasions, when I have revealed this information about my daughter, I have been met with understanding or asked for advice. When our cleaning lady learned about Camille's sexual orientation, she asked me, 'Would you agree to speak to a friend of mine? You see, she recently learned her only son is gay. She is devastated.'

I said, 'Tell her that her son already faces tons of rejection. She should ask herself if she wants to be another person rejecting him or if she wants to be a supportive, loving mother offering a safe space for him.'

Many parents feel disappointed when they discover their child's same-sex attraction. Many grieve for an image of their child that was fabricated in their minds and was, in fact, wrong all along. However, the revelation of a child's genuine sexual orientation can actually bring parents closer to their child, as it's an opportunity to know their identity better.

Li Hua's comments provoke a debate inside my head. What is my public responsibility as a mother of a lesbian daughter? Do I have one beyond protecting and supporting her as an individual? I had, until now, never thought of this. Yet I realise that I do care to change hearts and minds and to contribute to a society that is open and inclusive, both for my daughter and for any other discriminated minority. I tell myself this means I should seize opportunities to be outspoken and to be a conscientious supporter. Am I already outspoken enough, though? And, most importantly, how open does Camille want me to be? Ultimately, I am sharing information about her. At this point, I make a plan to ask her.

I arrive home, drop my massaged body in the hammock and text Camille about the incident. I finish with a question, 'Should I have answered with the truthful, but incomplete answer, "Camille still doesn't have a boyfriend?" or should I use the occasion to sensitise?'

And then comes Camille's answer.

'My feeling is, if people don't ask correctly, they don't deserve the full truth. Even less a personal answer. When I am asked if I have a boyfriend, I almost always answer with a simple no. Only when asked if I have a partner do I offer a full response. And, as a survival rule, I never share this information when at the hairdresser or the aesthetician. It's a safe bet, and maybe I exaggerate, but I don't want to be in that awkward silence you mentioned. I prefer not to reveal it because it reminds me every time that the battle is not won and that there is still much to do.

'But I refuse to hide. I will walk chin up with A's hand in mine on the street. I do it in support of gay boys and girls. The comments we receive in the street are sexist and dehumanising, but I will not stop holding her hand and neither will she stop holding mine. It's true that I am not interested in educating people. At times I try, but I get tired of it. Fortunately, there are others who do it more openly and are more engaged. We are all fighting our battles.

'Oh, and of course Li Hua has asked me many times if I have a boyfriend. I've always said no. And now I know I won't go to her again for a massage. I know the silence you are talking about. I don't want to experience it.'

Li Hua's homophobic reaction has sparked a reflection on my public advocacy. I am proud of my daughter and her determination. I stand by her. This is part of who she is and I now realise I want to say it publicly to whoever cares to listen *and* whoever doesn't. I celebrate the diversity that Camille has brought to our family; she has enriched our lives, our perspectives, and our understanding of gender and sexual orientation.

I will not avoid the topic precisely because it is still a taboo for many. I will speak up because I can. It's easier for me to speak because I am not the person experiencing rejection.

I stand up for my daughter's right to live a full, free, self-determined life independent of her sexual orientation. From now on, I tell myself, I'll be a more deliberate and outspoken advocate for diversity, visibility, affirmation, and inclusion.

Prejudice won't vanish because we keep it under wraps. I will be more alert to homophobia and will seek to dismantle it whenever I encounter it. I will not demonise the homophobe, so I will return to Li Hua, and when I have the occasion, I will try to persuade her that same-sex attraction is not a disease.

For Camille

Blow Jobs Suck

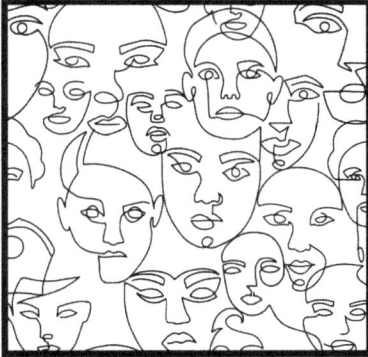

BLOW JOBS SUCK

By Anne Belford

It is a truth universally acknowledged that a man in possession of a penis must be in want of a blow job. And yet, one fact remains, one obvious fact so blatantly ignored that sometimes I wonder if I'm the only woman on earth aware of it. Much like in *The Emperor's New Clothes*, could I be the only one who sees that the king is naked?

Look, men pee through the same fleshy device they ask us to put into our mouths.

Let that sink in.

Would I lick a urinal? The answer is no, but if I wrap my precious lips around a penis, isn't that almost the same thing – especially if said penis hasn't been washed before the deed? And when your partner reaches the throes of his passion and bursts in ecstasy inside your mouth, don't you ever wonder if some droplets of pee came along for the ride?

Because I totally do.

Men sweat, all right? Their balls sweat, their ass crack sweats, and when you put a penis in your mouth, you better believe it will taste like his sweat made love to a fart. It always does.

One time during a girls' night out, a friend showed me a dick pic from one of her hook ups. 'It's such a beautiful penis,' she said proudly. 'I want to suck it all the time.'

Okay, look. As far as penises went, this guy's was quite nice. I'll admit it. His dick was hairless, smooth, and just the right size. I can appreciate a pretty penis like everyone else, but just because something is pretty doesn't mean I want it in my mouth. Penises, pretty or ugly, old or new, always taste like farts. Except, of course, when the guy showers right before the deed. Then the penis tastes like soap with a light tinge of fart, which is better, but honestly, not enough to motivate me.

And their happy discharge? Ew. Just ew. Are we supposed to pretend it tastes like the most delicious nectar of the gods? Newsflash: it doesn't. It's warm, sticky, and between you and me, I've never had it in my mouth long enough to actually taste it.

Spit that shit on his belly, girlfriend. You've done your duty.

I'll never forget the poor sap who once, after releasing the throes of his passion into my poor mouth, looked down at me, smiled, and asked, 'Did you cum, too, babe?'

No, buddy. Not even close.

On that note, don't even get me started on pacing. Some men think women (and other men, of course) don't have gag reflexes and therefore viciously ram their little beasts into our throats, thinking we're actually enjoying that.

Why? *Why?*

Dear reader, rest assured there's a special place in hell for such men. Blow jobs suck, but deep throating is just, well, gag-inducing. Literally.

Seriously, how can anyone think that being suffocated by a penis, in what can only be described as a near-death experience, is something a person might enjoy?

So, men: *maybe* don't use our mouths like a back-alley glory hole? *Maybe* wash your little partner down there? That would really make the job easier. But would it make it enjoyable? It depends.

Some may argue that they feel empowered in owning their partner's pleasure so completely and I can respect that. Actually, I would also like that in theory, but not everything that sounds good in theory is good in real life. Take pigs flying, for example. The theory would be awesome (flying bacon), but in real life, you'd get bombed by pig shit every five minutes and that's just not worth the cost.

One might also argue that going down on a lady is not the most pleasant of experiences, to which I say: well, duh! We sweat too. It smells like a fish market down there, people.

I wouldn't go down on myself, so why should you?

And let's be honest: there's no way you won't get some lost droplet of pee on your tongue. Just saying. In fact, I wouldn't wish that upon my worst enemy, but to be fair, I would wish someone deep throated them instead, because that's 100 percent worse and my enemies must pay in coin and tears.

I think going down on a lady is equally disgusting to blow-ing a guy, because you know, equality. Also, between you and me, our lady parts smell a lot worse than theirs. Trust me, you do *not* want to go down on me after a yoga session.

In the end, it's also about being fair. Hence the reciprocity principle: you do me and I do you. Which is fine and dandy assuming both parties enjoy putting their mouths where they don't belong.

If you ask me, I prefer using mine to drink a fine Barolo wine and taste some delicious chocolate and fine cheese instead of sampling a smelly penis.

Here's a thought, and I know it's wildly shocking, but hear me out. Don't walk away, okay? Keep an open mind.

What if we kept the 'down under' under? What happens below the belt stays under the belt. What if, instead, we used our hands?

Seriously, they're easier to clean and you won't need a Tic Tac afterwards to mask the smell of dick coming out of your mouth. It might even be better for your neck. Plus, it's a win-win for those lazy days when you don't want to put in the effort.

Et voilà.

I'm Anne Belford, and I hope you've enjoyed my TED talk.

Nine True Facts About Hearts

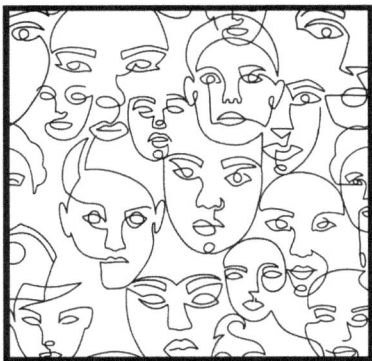

NINE TRUE FACTS ABOUT HEARTS

By Tai Farnsworth

1. Music changes your heartbeat. Your heartbeat is the same as an eighty-year-old man's because your music is from the 1950s. I grew up in prime mix-CD era, so I made you a Spotify playlist of all the songs I wanted you to hear. Which, of course, quickly morphed into a sappy, lovey, over-the-top collection of songs by bands that film their music videos barefoot in cliffside forests in the middle of thunderstorms. But when we were listening to the same song at the same time, I knew we were in sync. Our heartbeats slowed to match the music, to match each other. A love story in three minutes written just for us. Every lyric a poem from our book.

2. Your heart beats around 115,000 times a day. Obviously, it's not the same for everyone. Or for every day. For example, remember the night we went to a café to work? You had two different coloured highlighters and a pen in just one hand and

you flipped through pages of printouts rapidly making nota-tions. I thought I was reading, but mostly I was watching you. The freckles on your nose were a perfect surprise each time I looked at your face. Exactly as expected, yet still shocking. You were always like that – familiar but strange. We scuffed our toes over the gravel in the parking lot, feigning nervousness. We chain-smoked and talked about work and music. When you threw your butt on the ground, I lectured you about lit-tering, but you never stopped smiling. 'Will you just shut up?' you said, grabbing my face and pressing your lips to mine. We stood there, frozen in every potential, scared to move for-ward, our lips begging for answers. Right then, as the night drained from my body, my heart beat three times faster than normal. Running circles around my brain, racing through my veins, dancing in my stomach. That day my heart beat around 130,000 times. Every day with you.

3. The rhythm of the heart is maintained by an electrical system. I tell you this because I want you to know that every time we touched, I felt jolted alive. No, that's not quite right. It was more than that. Bigger. When you texted me 'Good morning, my beautiful evergreen,' my body tingled with the joy of it all. I felt the current of your heartbeat from miles away. Our electrical systems thrummed across the city, tan-gling, sparking a fire of passion inside of me. You told me my soul was silly, that you wanted to swallow me whole, that you missed my energy. You told me I was the most genuine, kind, understanding person you'd ever met. The bolt of each word pushed through the electrical system of your heart and right into mine.

4. Exercise is imperative to heart health. This is why I al-

ways wanted to fuck: I was worried about your heart health. Post-coital, lying in a sweaty mess on my cum-covered quilt, your heart would beat heavy on my stomach or back and I would think, 'Good, you're healthy.' It took so long for us to get there, but once we crossed that threshold, I couldn't stop tasting desire on my lips. Before the first time we had sex, I straddled you at the bar, my friends dancing dizzy around us, and kissed you hard, breathing my want into your mouth. My moans pulled something feral from you and you pushed me off your lap and grabbed my hand. 'Enough. Go to your car. Meet me at your house,' you said. We didn't even wave good-bye to my friends. The next morning, one of my housemates asked me how my night was, a laugh wrapped around her ciga-rette. Before I could answer, she said, 'Don't worry. I recorded it.' And she played a voice memo on her phone of me climax-ing with the words 'fuck' and 'god' and 'shit' spilling out of my mouth at two in the morning. That was when our hearts were the healthiest.

5. Your heart is about the size of a fist. Once you asked me to fuck you with my strap-on. You told me you wanted every part of me inside of you. And more. I was nervous, but you said we could go slow. *Maybe this is what straight people feel like when they lose their virginity*, you texted. We lit candles. We put on our playlist. Our hearts' rhythms merged. I allowed my mouth to travel the expanse of your body. Tasting every sweetness, every saltiness. When you begged me to fuck you, my own pussy became a throbbing ocean of desire. Want over-whelmed me. Every part of me needed to be inside you. And when you came, the rocking of your hips on top of me made me cum, too. But I wanted more. Hunger consumed me. I

needed you to consume me. On my knees, I opened myself to you. Offered myself to you. Two fingers, three fingers, more, everything. I was full of you. *Your heart is about the size of a fist*, I thought. *Your heart is inside me.*

6. Human lungs develop a little lopsided, the left lung smaller, to make room for your heart. How unsurprising that the heart is so powerful that the body builds itself around it. My body changed for loving you. My heart pumped with your name, shifting the molecules of my existence. Remember when your head was in my lap and I tied the waves of your hair around my fingers? That was when my heart re-wrote my story to include yours. That was when I told you I loved you, my hand covering your mouth. *Don't say it back, please,* I asked. *I want you to say it on your own. Without obligation.* I wanted you to wait till your heart was so overwhelmed with love for me that it changed each atom of your existence. I wanted your heart to be its most powerful self, pumping blood into your body that knew only love for me.

7. Heart cells stop dividing. This is why cancer of the heart is so rare. It's also probably why your heart was never big enough to share. Once your heart was built around someone else, I never really stood a chance. You couldn't evolve to have me in your life; your heart was already formed, made without my name in its walls. Sometimes we'd be sitting in the dark watching the cherries of our cigarettes light up the night and she'd call. You would answer. You always answered her call. My heart would beat truths into the night. *She isn't meant for you. She loves someone else.* But the worst was when you'd leave to be with her. And I let you because I thought if I gave you time, you'd eventually see how much happier your heart

would be if it was with mine. You didn't. Your heart cells weren't dividing anymore.

8. Broken hearts feel similar to heart attacks. I know this because I've had a broken heart. More than once. The one you created was particularly calamitous because my heart was still barely healed from the previous break. Every night before that last night, we lay wrapped in each other and you held my hand while I walked you through all my rainy days. I cut a window into my chest so I could show you the stitches on my heart. *They were fools*, you said. *Only a fool would hurt you.* And yet, I stood across from you, scuffing my foot in disbelief, long since past my nervousness, and you detailed all your lies. Your words ripped through the scabs I'd spent almost a year building. Turns out you were never trying to hold my heart in your hand. This wasn't about building for you, this was about distracting. This was a journey of mending your own broken heart with pieces of mine. A shattering of hearts that left me sobbing smoke into the night air. *We are fools,* I thought.

9. The heart can continue beating even when it's disconnected from the body. This is true and verifiable by science. I'm also an expert because I walked away from you that night and felt my heart ripping itself from my body. I held my heart in my hands, felt its dull, listless throbbing, and waited for it to still. For days I was sure it would stop beating. Out of respect for my heart and our many years together, I tried to make its last days pleasant. To keep lint from gathering on my heart's aorta or pulmonary artery, I put it in a Ziploc bag. But I didn't want my heart to feel like I was treating it clinically, so I put the Ziploc in a small velvet purse around my wrist. I walked around with my hand on my chest, keeping my

heart near its home, offering it as much comfort as I could. At night, under my covers, I held my heart close to my mouth and whispered words of kindness that it had forgotten it deserved. *You are good. You are powerful in your softness. Don't give up all your tender beauty.* My heart stitched up its wounds and kept beating, looking for a future love song to sync up to. But it refused to go back into my chest, knowing the safety my skin and muscle and ribs offered was insufficient. So I keep my heart in that bag around my wrist always, showing the world my unending tender beauty, giving it all my softness. Here, can't you see? Watch it beat.

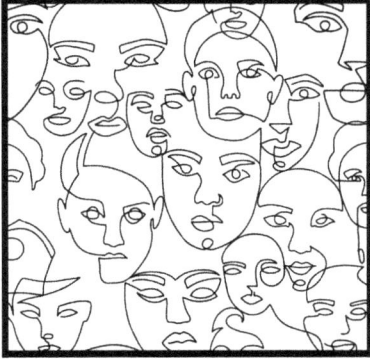

Afterword

This project has been built on a foundation of love: love for ourselves, for each other, and for our flaws as humans. We are grateful to everyone who shared in this project with us.

We would especially like to thank:

Our own loved ones, for giving us the space to build this book;

Laura Burge, editor extraordinaire;

Chris Allen, for our stunning cover design;

The authors who were courageous enough to send us their deeply personal stories;

The Zurich writing community, and particularly Jill and Clara for their time and advice.

Thank you all.